# BLOOD GLUCOSE CONTROL SOLUTION

*The Ultimate Guide to Balance Blood sugar with proven method, support supplement, recipes, and diets*

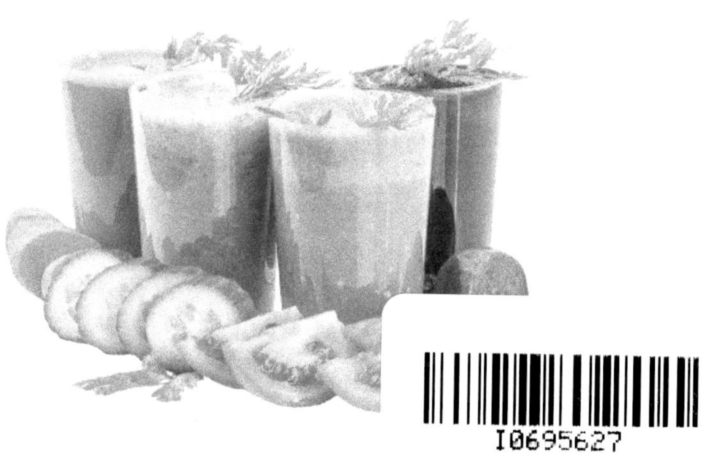



**Dr. Ryan K. McNutt**

# Copyright © by Ryan K. McNutt 2023.

# TABLE OF CONTENT

# INTRODUCTION

There lived a man named David who had been struggling with high blood sugar for over 4 years. Despite his best efforts, his glucose levels remained stubbornly high, and he had to rely on medication to keep them in check.

Frustrated and determined to find an alternative solution, he embarked on a journey to explore the potential of dietary supplements.

David began his quest for better blood sugar management which led him to so some of my posts on Facebook. After going through the article, he realized that proper supplements can be used to manage blood sugar then he clicked through the link and purchased this book to help him regulate blood sugar.

With the guidance from this book, David started incorporating these supplements into his daily routine. He meticulously monitored his blood sugar levels and tracked his progress over several months. To his surprise and delight, David began to notice positive changes.

His glucose readings gradually improved, and he felt more energetic throughout the day. As his confidence grew, he became even more dedicated to his supplement regimen, ensuring he took them consistently alongside his well-balanced diet and regular exercise routine in this book.

Over time, David's hard work paid off. His blood sugar levels became stable within a healthy range, and he no longer needed as much medication.

His doctor was impressed by the progress and eventually adjusted his treatment plan to reflect the improvements.

David's commitment to his health and the use of carefully selected supplements made a significant difference in his life.

Feeling healthier than he had in years, David continued to maintain his lifestyle changes. He shared his success story with friends and family, emphasizing the importance of consulting with healthcare professionals before starting any supplement regimen.

His journey became an inspiration for those facing similar challenges, showing them that with the right guidance and determination, it was possible to take control of their blood sugar naturally.

David's story became a testament to the potential of supplements as part of a comprehensive approach to blood sugar management.

It reminded everyone that while supplements could be helpful, they were most effective when combined with a balanced diet, exercise, and regular medical guidance. With perseverance and the right tools.

In the intricate symphony of human health, few elements play as pivotal a role as blood sugar. It is the life-sustaining conductor of our metabolic orchestra, orchestrating the energy flow that powers our bodies. Yet, like a double-edged sword, blood sugar can be both a source of vitality and a harbinger of havoc when its delicate balance is disrupted.

The term "blood sugar" refers to the concentration of glucose, a simple sugar, circulating in our bloodstream.

This seemingly mundane substance is the fuel that propels our cells, enabling them to carry out their myriad functions, from muscle contractions to brain activity.

But, it's not just about energy; blood sugar has profound implications for our overall health.

The equilibrium of blood sugar is a precarious one, akin to a tightrope walk between sustenance and chaos. Too high, and it can ravage our arteries, nerves, and organs, leaving a trail of devastation in the form of diabetes and its far-reaching complications.

Too low, and it plunges us into a state of trembling weakness, cognitive impairment, and if left unaddressed, unconsciousness.

Our modern lifestyles, characterized by sedentary habits and diets laden with refined sugars, have tipped the scales towards chronic hyperglycemia, contributing to a global epidemic of diabetes and metabolic disorders.

Conversely, the fear of plummeting blood sugar levels has driven many to compulsively monitor their intake, often at the cost of their mental and emotional well-being.

In this intricate dance of glucose, insulin, and cells, understanding the profound impact of blood sugar on health is not just a matter of academic interest; it's a matter of life and vitality.

In the pages that follow, we will explore the multifaceted dimensions of blood sugar, from its regulation to its implications for various aspects of our well-being.

So, join us on this journey through the corridors of your own metabolic symphony, as we unravel the intricate interplay of blood sugar and health.

Blood sugar control is vital for both preventing and managing various health conditions, improving overall quality of life, and promoting long-term health and well-being.

It is essential to adopt a healthy lifestyle, including a balanced diet, regular physical activity recommended in this book, to achieve and maintain optimal blood sugar control.

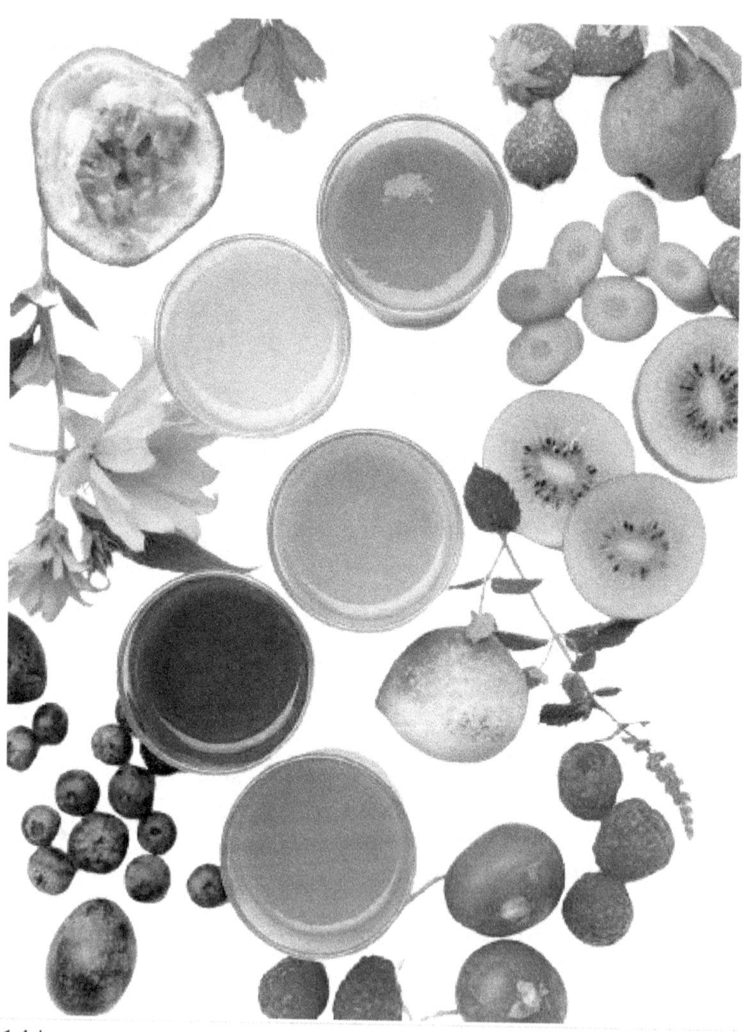

# CHAPTER 1

## The Basics of Blood Sugar

Blood sugar, scientifically known as glucose, serves as the primary energy source for our bodies. Its regulation is a remarkably intricate process, crucial for maintaining overall health. In this comprehensive exploration, we will delve into the mechanisms behind blood sugar regulation, the various types of sugars, and their effects on our physiology.

The human body employs a sophisticated system to regulate blood sugar levels, ensuring they remain within a narrow range. This orchestration primarily revolves around two key hormones: insulin and glucagon.

**Insulin:** When you consume carbohydrates, your digestive system breaks them down into glucose, causing your blood sugar levels to rise. To counteract this increase, the pancreas, a gland located behind your stomach, secretes insulin into the bloodstream. Think of insulin as the gatekeeper; it allows glucose to enter cells, where it can be used for immediate energy or stored as glycogen in the liver and muscles for later use. This insulin-driven process efficiently lowers blood sugar levels, preserving stability.

**Glucagon:** When blood sugar levels fall, as they do during fasting or physical activity, the pancreas releases another hormone known as glucagon. Glucagon serves as an antidote to insulin.

It causes the liver to convert glycogen stored in the liver into glucose, which is then released into the bloodstream. This process raises blood sugar levels, supplying cells with the energy they require.

# An Overview of Sugar Types

Sugars are not all created equal, and their effects on blood sugar levels vary. Let's look at the different forms of sugars and their effects:

**1. Monosaccharides and disaccharides (simple sugars)**

a. Glucose: Also known as "blood sugar," glucose is a monosaccharide found in a variety of foods such as fruits and honey. It is quickly absorbed into the bloodstream, resulting in a significant rise in blood sugar levels.

b. Fructose: Another monosaccharide found naturally in fruits, vegetables, and honey.

While it does not immediately elevate blood sugar levels like glucose, it can lead to a variety of health issues, including fatty liver disease.

c. Sucrose: Sucrose, often known as table sugar, is a disaccharide made up of equal parts glucose and fructose. During digestion, it is swiftly broken down into its constituent sugars, causing a surge in blood sugar.

## 2. Polysaccharides (Complex Carbohydrates)

a. Starch: A complex carbohydrate composed of long chains of glucose molecules. Starch-rich foods, such as potatoes, rice, and cereals, must be digested in order to be broken down into individual glucose units for absorption. When compared to simple sugars, this results in a more gradual and persistent increase in blood sugar levels.

b. Fiber: Although it is not a sugar, dietary fiber is important in blood sugar management.

Soluble fiber, found in foods such as oats and lentils, can assist in stabilizing blood sugar levels by slowing the absorption of glucose.

## Possible Causes of Abnormal Blood Sugar Levels

A multitude of events can cause abnormal blood sugar levels, which can be either too high (hyperglycemia) or too low (hypoglycemia). Here are some of the possible causes of high blood sugar:

**Hyperglycemia (High Blood Sugar)**

1. Diabetes: Hyperglycemia is a hallmark of both type 1 and type 2 diabetes. In type 1 diabetes, the body doesn't produce insulin, while in type 2 diabetes, the body either doesn't use insulin effectively or doesn't produce enough.

2. Diet: Consuming excessive carbohydrates, especially sugary and refined foods, can cause a rapid spike in blood sugar levels.

3. Lack of Physical Activity: Physical activity helps regulate blood sugar. Sedentism can result in elevated blood sugar levels.

4. Stress: Stress hormones can cause blood sugar levels to rise. This is commonly known as "stress-induced hyperglycemia."

5. Illness or Infection: Infections and illnesses can lead to higher blood sugar levels as the body's immune response releases stress hormones.

6. Certain Medications: Some medications, such as steroids and certain antipsychotic drugs, can cause hyperglycemia as a side effect.

**Hypoglycemia (Low Blood Sugar)**

1. Diabetes Medications: Excessive use or improper dosing of insulin or oral diabetes medications can lead to hypoglycemia.

2. Skipping Meals: Not eating regular meals or snacks, especially for individuals taking diabetes medications, can result in low blood sugar.

3. Excessive Alcohol Consumption: Alcohol can interfere with the liver's ability to release stored glucose, leading to hypoglycemia.

4. Increased Physical Activity: Strenuous exercise without proper adjustments to insulin or food intake can cause low blood sugar.

5. Medical Conditions: Certain medical conditions, such as adrenal insufficiency or hypothyroidism, can lead to low blood sugar.

6. Tumor or Insulinoma: Rarely, tumors of the pancreas called insulinomas can cause excess insulin production, leading to hypoglycemia.

7. Overdose of Diabetes Medications: In cases of accidental or deliberate overdose of diabetes medications, hypoglycemia can occur.

It's essential to monitor blood sugar levels regularly, especially for individuals with diabetes or those at risk for abnormal blood sugar levels.

Consult with a healthcare provider if you experience persistent high or low blood sugar levels to determine the underlying cause and develop an appropriate management plan.

# Effects of Abnormal Blood Sugar Levels

Abnormal blood sugar levels, whether they are too high (hyperglycemia) or too low (hypoglycemia), can have significant and sometimes severe effects on the human body. Maintaining blood sugar levels within a narrow range is essential for overall health and well-being. Here are some of the key effects of abnormal blood sugar levels:

1. **Hyperglycemia (High Blood Sugar):**

- Increased Thirst and Urination: When blood sugar levels are elevated, the body tries to get rid of the excess glucose through urine, leading to increased thirst and frequent urination.

- Fatigue: Cells may not get the energy they need, causing fatigue and weakness.

- Blurry Vision: High blood sugar levels can affect the fluid balance in the eye, leading to blurred vision.

- Weight Loss: In some cases, hyperglycemia can lead to unintentional weight loss as the body breaks down fat and muscle for energy.

- Increased Infections: High sugar levels can weaken the immune system, making individuals more susceptible to infections.

- Long-term Complications: Prolonged hyperglycemia can result in serious complications such as cardiovascular disease, kidney damage, nerve damage (neuropathy), and eye problems (retinopathy).

## 2. Hypoglycemia (Low Blood Sugar):

- Confusion and Irritability: Low blood sugar levels can affect cognitive function, leading to confusion, irritability, and difficulty concentrating.

- Shakiness and Sweating: Hypoglycemia often causes trembling and excessive sweating.

- Rapid Heartbeat: The body releases adrenaline in response to low blood sugar, which can increase heart rate.

- Hunger: A strong sense of hunger, even if you've recently eaten, is common during hypoglycemic episodes.

- Severe Hypoglycemia: In severe cases, hypoglycemia can lead to seizures and unconsciousness, and, if left untreated, it can be life-threatening.

3. Impaired Cognitive Function: Both high and low blood sugar levels can impair cognitive function. Chronically elevated blood sugar levels are associated with a higher risk of cognitive decline and conditions like dementia.

4. Mood Changes: Blood sugar fluctuations can also impact mood. High blood sugar levels may lead to irritability and mood swings, while low blood sugar can cause feelings of anxiety and even depression.

5. Cardiovascular Effects: Prolonged hyperglycemia can damage blood vessels and increase the risk of heart disease, stroke, and hypertension.

6. Nerve Damage: High blood sugar levels can damage nerves, leading to neuropathy, which can cause pain, tingling, and numbness in the extremities.

7. Vision Problems: Elevated blood sugar levels can damage the blood vessels in the eyes, potentially leading to diabetic retinopathy and vision loss.

8. Kidney Damage: Diabetes and consistently high blood sugar levels can damage the kidneys over time, potentially leading to kidney disease and the need for dialysis or transplantation.

9. Foot Problems: High blood sugar can lead to poor circulation and nerve damage in the feet, increasing the risk of foot ulcers and amputations.

It's crucial for individuals with diabetes or those at risk of blood sugar abnormalities to manage their condition carefully through lifestyle changes, medication, or insulin therapy as prescribed by healthcare professionals.

Regular monitoring of blood sugar levels and maintaining a healthy diet, regular exercise, and stress management can help prevent these adverse effects and promote overall well-being. Early intervention and effective management are key to reducing the risks associated with abnormal blood sugar levels.

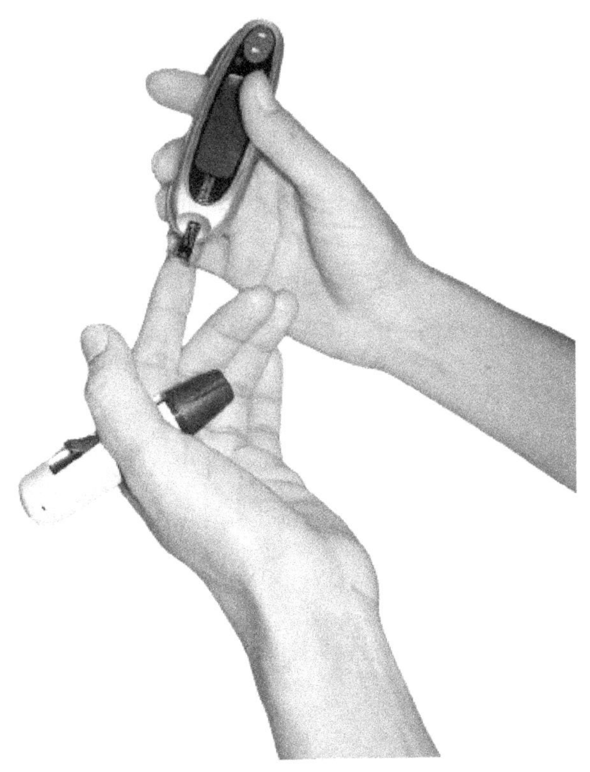

# CHAPTER 2

# Assessing Your Current Health

Monitoring and maintaining healthy blood sugar levels is essential for overall well-being, particularly for individuals at risk of or already managing conditions like diabetes. Self-assessment tools can be invaluable in helping you gauge your current health status and track changes in your blood sugar levels over time. In this detailed exploration, we will discuss the importance of self-assessment tools for blood sugar, the various methods available, and how to use them effectively.

**Why Self-Assessment Tools for Blood Sugar Matter:**

1. Early Detection: Self-assessment tools allow for the early detection of abnormal blood sugar levels. Catching potential issues in their early stages can be critical in preventing or managing conditions like prediabetes or diabetes.

2. Monitoring Progress: If you are already managing your blood sugar, self-assessment tools provide a way to track your progress.

They help you understand the effectiveness of lifestyle changes, dietary adjustments, or medications.

3. Personalized Insights: Self-assessment tools can provide personalized insights into how your body responds to various factors like diet, exercise, stress, and sleep. This information enables you to make informed decisions about your health.

4. Empowerment: By actively participating in monitoring your blood sugar, you take a proactive role in your health. This sense of empowerment can lead to better adherence to treatment plans and healthier lifestyle choices.

## Types of Self-Assessment Tools for Blood Sugar

1. Blood Glucose Monitors (Glucometers): Glucometers are portable devices that measure your blood sugar levels at a given moment. To use them, you typically prick your finger to obtain a small blood sample, which is then analyzed by the device. These tools are widely used by individuals with diabetes for daily monitoring.

2. Continuous Glucose Monitoring (CGM) Systems: CGM systems use a tiny sensor implanted under the skin to deliver real-time data on blood sugar levels.

They continually monitor glucose levels throughout the day, providing a detailed picture of trends and changes. CGM devices are especially beneficial for diabetics since they can provide insight into how specific diets, activities, or stress affect blood sugar levels.

3. HbA1c (Hemoglobin A1c) Tests: This blood test examines your blood sugar levels throughout the previous two to three months. It provides a more thorough assessment of your total blood sugar control and is frequently used by healthcare experts to assess long-term treatment.

4. Urine Glucose Testing Strips: Although less widely used nowadays, these strips can provide a basic indication of blood sugar levels. They function by determining the amount of glucose discharged in the urine. They are, however, less exact than blood-based approaches.

# How to Effectively Use Self-Assessment Tools:

1. Obey Instructions: When using a glucometer, CGM system, or other equipment, it's critical to strictly adhere to the manufacturer's instructions. Accurate outcomes are ensured by proper procedure.

2. Establish a Routine: When it comes to blood sugar monitoring, consistency is essential. Set up a regimen for testing or utilizing CGM systems and attempt to keep to it as much as possible.

3. Keep Track of Your Data: Keep track of your blood sugar levels. Take note of the time and date, as well as any pertinent factors such as meals, exercise, stress, or medicine dosages. This data can assist you and your healthcare provider in identifying patterns and making educated decisions.

4. develop Target Ranges: Collaborate with your healthcare team to develop target blood sugar ranges that are

appropriate for your specific health goals and conditions. These goals will direct your self-evaluation efforts.

5. Interpret the Results: Know what your blood sugar levels signify. If you have diabetes or prediabetes, your doctor will help you understand the results and make any required changes to your treatment plan.

6. Seek Professional Advice: Self-assessment tools are useful, but they should be used in addition to, not in instead of, frequent healthcare visits. Discuss your findings with your healthcare physician, resolve any concerns, and make any required changes to your diabetes treatment plan.

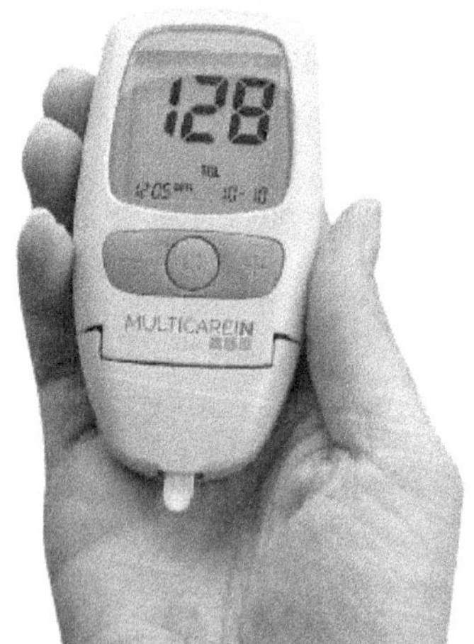

# CHAPTER 3

# Blood Sugar Support Supplements

Blood sugar support supplements are intended to help individuals with diabetes or those at risk of blood sugar fluctuations regulate and maintain appropriate blood sugar levels. These supplements frequently include a combination of natural compounds such as chromium, berberine, cinnamon, and alpha-lipoic acid, which have been examined for their ability to improve insulin sensitivity, increase glucose uptake by cells, and decrease sugar absorption from the digestive tract. Blood sugar support supplements attempt to improve the efficiency of insulin and promote improved glucose utilization by giving the body these specific nutrients and bioactive substances, ultimately helping to stabilize blood sugar levels. However, it is crucial to remember that these supplements should not be used in place of a healthy diet, exercise, and any prescribed medications, but rather as part of a complete strategy for blood sugar management.

Individuals thinking about using such supplements should contact a healthcare expert to establish their suitability and dosages.

Typically, blood sugar support supplements act through multiple mechanisms:

1. Improving Insulin Sensitivity: Many of these supplements contain substances such as chromium and alpha-lipoic acid, which can aid with insulin sensitivity. This implies that the body's response to the insulin it generates improves, allowing cells to absorb glucose more effectively.

2. Sugar Absorption Reduction: Some supplements, such as berberine and gymnema sylvestre, have been demonstrated to decrease sugar absorption in the intestines. They can help reduce fast rises in blood sugar levels after meals by doing so.

3. Increasing Glucose Uptake: Certain chemicals in these supplements, such as cinnamon extract, can increase cellular glucose uptake. This means that cells can utilize glucose for energy more efficiently.

4. Anti-Inflammatory Effects: Insulin resistance and blood sugar abnormalities can be exacerbated by chronic inflammation. Some supplements, such as curcumin (found in turmeric), have anti-inflammatory qualities that may help with blood sugar control.

5. Antioxidant Properties: Antioxidants found in these supplements, such as alpha-lipoic acid and vitamin C, can help protect cells from oxidative stress, which can contribute to diabetes issues.

6. Balancing Hormones: Certain supplements may assist in regulating hormones related to blood sugar regulation. For example, bitter melon extract has been studied for its potential to affect insulin production.

It's vital to remember that the effectiveness of blood sugar support supplements could differ from person to person, and they are most useful when used as part of a comprehensive strategy for blood sugar management.

A nutritious diet, regular exercise, correct medication (if needed), and contact with a healthcare practitioner are all critical components of maintaining stable blood sugar levels. Individuals interested in using these supplements should connect with a healthcare provider to establish the most suited selections and dosages based on their unique needs and situations.

There are many blood sugar support supplements available on the market, each with its specific combination of components and mechanisms of action. When studying these supplements, it's vital to grasp their primary parameters to make an informed choice for regulating blood sugar successfully.

Here are some common blood sugar support supplements and the important aspects to consider for each:

## 1. Cinnamon Extract:

Cinnamon extract supplements usually contain bioactive compounds, including Cinnamaldehyde, renowned for its potential to increase insulin sensitivity and promote glucose uptake by cells.

- Dosage: Typically, doses range from 500 mg to 2,000 mg daily, however, it's vital to follow the product's recommended dosage.

## 2. Berberine:

Berberine is derived from numerous plants and has shown the potential to decrease sugar absorption from the stomach and enhance insulin sensitivity.

- Dosage: Standard dosages vary from 500 mg to 1,500 mg daily, often divided into two or three doses each day.

## 3. Alpha-Lipoic Acid:

Alpha-lipoic acid is an antioxidant that may help reduce oxidative stress and promote insulin sensitivity.

- Dosage: Common doses are between 300 mg to 600 mg daily.

## 4. Gymnema Sylvestre:

Gymnema Sylvestre has been researched for its ability to lessen sugar absorption and cravings by blocking sugar receptors on the taste buds.

- Dosage: Typical dosages vary from 200 mg to 400 mg daily.

## 5. Chromium:

Chromium is a trace mineral that can increase insulin sensitivity and support glucose metabolism.

- Dosage: Common doses are in the range of 200 mcg to 1,000 mcg daily, although individual requirements may vary.

## 6. Bitter Melon Extract:

Bitter melon extract comprises compounds that may help regulate blood sugar via modulating insulin production.

- Dosage: Dosages generally range from 500 mg to 1,500 mg daily, however, it's crucial to follow the product's directions.

## 7. Fenugreek Seed Extract:

Fenugreek seeds have soluble fiber and compounds that may help lower blood sugar levels and boost insulin sensitivity.

- Dosage: Common doses vary from 500 mg to 1,500 mg daily.

## 8. Turmeric (Curcumin):

Curcumin, the major element in turmeric, has anti-inflammatory and antioxidant qualities that can aid overall health, including blood sugar regulation.

- Dosage: Depending on the product, dosing may vary, but normal amounts range from 500 mg to 2,000 mg daily.

## 9. Magnesium:

Magnesium is a mineral that performs a crucial function in glucose metabolism and insulin sensitivity.

- Dosage: Dosage recommendations may vary, but normal doses range from 200 mg to 400 mg daily.

## 10. Vitamin D:

Vitamin D is vital for overall health, and its lack has been related to insulin resistance.

- Dosage: Dosages vary greatly, but a normal daily dose is 1,000 IU to 2,000 IU.

When considering blood sugar support supplements, it's essential to consult with a healthcare professional, especially if you have diabetes or are taking medication, as these supplements can interact with existing treatments. Additionally, individual responses to supplements may vary, so it's crucial to monitor your blood sugar levels and adjust your regimen as needed under the guidance of a healthcare provider. A holistic approach that includes a balanced diet, regular exercise, stress management, and appropriate medical care should always be at the forefront of blood sugar management.

## Combining Supplements for Synergy

Combining supplements for synergy in blood sugar management can be an effective approach for individuals looking to optimize their glycemic control. This strategy involves carefully selecting and combining supplements with complementary mechanisms of action to achieve a more comprehensive and balanced approach to blood sugar regulation.

Here, we'll explore how this synergy works and the considerations to keep in mind.

## Mechanisms of Synergy:

Combining supplements for blood sugar management aims to address multiple aspects of glucose regulation simultaneously. For example, one supplement may focus on enhancing insulin sensitivity, while another may target reducing sugar absorption from the gut or reducing oxidative stress.

By using supplements with distinct mechanisms of action, you create a multifaceted approach that can provide more comprehensive support for blood sugar levels.

## Complementary Ingredients

Choosing supplements with complementary ingredients is key to achieving synergy. For instance, cinnamon extract and berberine can complement each other, as cinnamon may improve insulin sensitivity, while berberine can reduce sugar absorption from the intestines.

Similarly, combining alpha-lipoic acid, which has antioxidant properties, with gymnema sylvestre, known for its potential to reduce sugar cravings, can create a well-rounded strategy for blood sugar management.

## Balanced Dosages

When combining supplements, it's crucial to pay attention to dosages. Some supplements may have overlapping effects, so it's essential not to exceed recommended daily doses, as excessive intake can lead to adverse effects. Consulting with a healthcare professional or a registered dietitian is advisable to determine the appropriate dosages based on individual needs and specific health conditions.

## Monitoring and Adjustments

Regular monitoring of blood sugar levels is essential when combining supplements. This allows you to assess the effectiveness of the regimen and make necessary adjustments. Keep in mind that individual responses may vary, so it's vital to work closely with a healthcare provider to fine-tune the supplement regimen for optimal results.

## Safety and Interactions:

Safety is paramount when combining supplements. Some supplements may interact with medications or have contraindications for certain medical conditions. Therefore, it's crucial to disclose all supplements you are taking to your healthcare provider to ensure they are safe and compatible with your current treatment plan.

## Holistic Approach:

While combining supplements can be a valuable component of blood sugar management, it should be integrated into a holistic approach. A balanced diet that includes complex carbohydrates, fiber, and healthy fats, along with regular physical activity and stress management, plays a vital role in maintaining stable blood sugar levels. Medications, if prescribed, should also be taken as directed.

# Choosing the Right Blood Sugar Support Supplements

Choosing the right blood sugar support supplements is crucial for managing your blood glucose levels effectively, especially if you have diabetes or are at risk of developing it. Here are some important factors to consider when selecting these supplements:

## 1. Consult with a Healthcare Professional

Before adding any blood sugar support supplements to your routine, consult with your healthcare provider or a registered dietitian. They can assess your individual health needs, current medications, and any potential interactions with supplements.

## 2. Check for Scientific Evidence

Look for supplements that have been scientifically studied and shown to be effective in supporting healthy blood sugar levels. Peer-reviewed research and clinical trials are excellent indicators of a supplement's reliability.

## 3. Read the Label

Carefully review the supplement's label to understand its ingredients. Look for key components like:

- Chromium: Helps with insulin sensitivity.

- Cinnamon: May help reduce blood sugar levels.

- Berberine: Supports glucose metabolism.

- Alpha-Lipoic Acid: A powerful antioxidant.

- Bitter Melon: May enhance insulin function.

- Gymnema Sylvestre: Helps reduce sugar cravings.

- Magnesium: Supports insulin action.

- Vitamins (e.g., B-complex): Play a role in glucose metabolism.

Avoid supplements with excessive fillers, artificial additives, or unnecessary ingredients.

## 4. Dosage and Form:

Pay attention to the recommended dosage and the form of the supplement (capsules, tablets, powder, etc.). Ensure that the dosage aligns with your specific needs and that the form is convenient for you to take.

## 5. Quality and Safety:

Choose supplements from reputable brands that adhere to good manufacturing practices (GMP) and have third-party testing for quality and purity. Look for certifications from organizations like the US Pharmacopeia (USP) or ConsumerLab.

## 6. Consider Your Diet:

Supplements should supplement, not replace, a healthy diet. Prioritize a healthy diet rich in whole grains, lean proteins, fruits, vegetables, and healthy fats. Supplements should be viewed as a supplement to your diet and not a substitute.

## 7. Monitor Blood Sugar Levels:

Monitor your blood sugar levels on a regular basis, as directed by your healthcare practitioner.

This will help you assess the effectiveness of the supplements and make necessary adjustments.

## 8. Be Cautious with Claims:

Be skeptical of supplements that promise miraculous results or quick fixes. Blood sugar management is a complex process, and supplements alone are unlikely to replace proper diet and lifestyle changes.

## 9. Consider Potential Interactions:

Some supplements may interact with the medications you are currently taking. Inform your healthcare provider of all supplements you plan to use to avoid any adverse interactions.

## 10. Track Your Progress:

Keep a journal to track how the supplement affects your blood sugar levels and overall well-being. This will help you and your healthcare provider make informed decisions about their continued use.

Remember that blood sugar support supplements should be part of a comprehensive approach to managing diabetes or blood sugar issues. They are not a standalone solution and should be used in conjunction with a healthy lifestyle, including a balanced diet and regular physical activity. Always seek professional guidance when making decisions about your health.

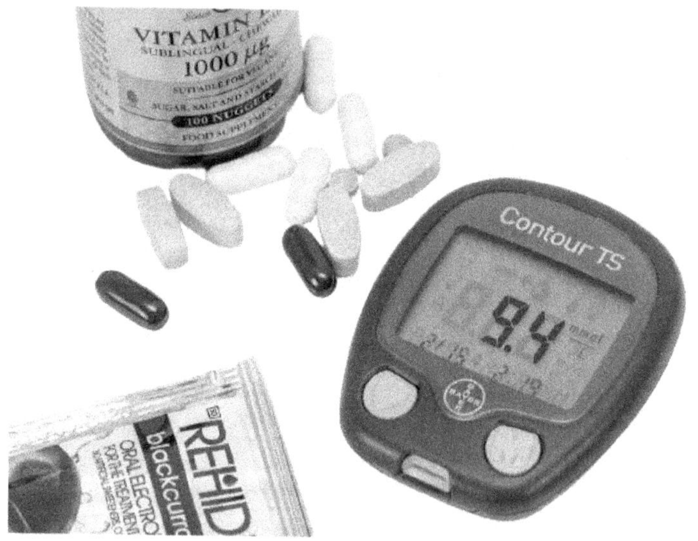

# CHAPTER 4

## The Blood Sugar Diet Plan

A balanced blood sugar diet is centered around principles that promote stable and healthy blood glucose levels. This dietary approach is of paramount importance for overall well-being, especially for individuals with diabetes or those at risk of developing it.

Here are the principles and the significance of adopting a balanced blood sugar diet:

1. Complex Carbohydrates: A balanced blood sugar diet emphasizes complex carbohydrates, such as whole grains (oats, quinoa, brown rice), legumes (beans, lentils), and vegetables. These carbohydrates are rich in fiber, which slows digestion and helps prevent rapid spikes in blood sugar levels after meals. The steady release of glucose provides sustained energy.

2. Portion Control: Controlling portion sizes is crucial for regulating blood sugar levels. Eating smaller, balanced

portions helps prevent excessive carbohydrate intake at one time, which can lead to blood sugar spikes.

3. Lean Proteins: Including lean protein sources like poultry, fish, tofu, and beans in your diet helps stabilize blood sugar levels. Protein slows down the absorption of carbohydrates, leading to more gradual increases in blood sugar after meals.

4. Healthy Fats: Incorporating healthy fats, such as avocados, nuts, seeds, and olive oil, into your diet helps improve insulin sensitivity and keeps blood sugar levels steady. These fats also provide essential nutrients for overall health.

5. Regular Meal Timing: Consistency in meal timing is crucial. Eating meals and snacks at regular intervals throughout the day can help maintain stable blood sugar levels. Skipping meals or going too long between meals can lead to blood sugar fluctuations.

6. Avoiding Sugary and Processed Foods: Limiting or avoiding foods and beverages high in added sugars, refined carbohydrates, and processed ingredients is essential.

These items can cause rapid spikes and crashes in blood sugar levels and contribute to insulin resistance.

7. Balanced Diet Planning: Consulting with a registered dietitian or healthcare provider to create a personalized meal plan tailored to your specific dietary needs and blood sugar goals can be highly beneficial. They can help you make informed choices and adjust your diet as needed.

8. Regular Monitoring: For individuals with diabetes or prediabetes, regular monitoring of blood sugar levels is essential to track progress and make necessary adjustments to the diet and medication if required.

9. Hydration: Staying well-hydrated is important for blood sugar control. Water helps transport glucose in the blood and supports overall metabolic processes.

10. Physical Activity: Incorporating regular physical activity into your routine can improve insulin sensitivity, making it easier for cells to absorb glucose from the bloodstream. This complements a balanced diet in managing blood sugar levels effectively.

The importance of a balanced blood sugar diet cannot be overstated. It helps prevent and manage diabetes, reduces the risk of complications associated with the condition, and promotes overall health and well-being.

Stable blood sugar levels can lead to increased energy, better mood, and a reduced risk of chronic diseases, making it a fundamental aspect of a healthy lifestyle. By adhering to these principles, individuals can take proactive steps to manage their blood sugar and improve their quality of life.

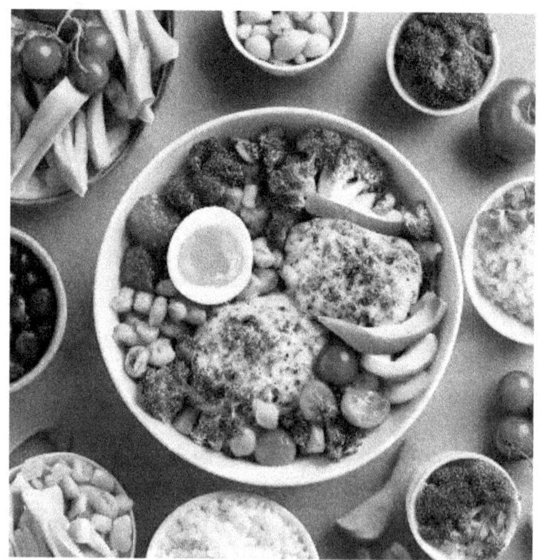

# 7-Day Blood Sugar Management Meal Plan with Detailed Recipes

Controlling blood sugar levels is critical for diabetics and those at risk of getting diabetes. A balanced meal plan can help regulate blood sugar levels.

Here's a 7-day meal plan that focuses on low-glycemic index foods, portion control, and balanced macronutrients to help with blood sugar control:

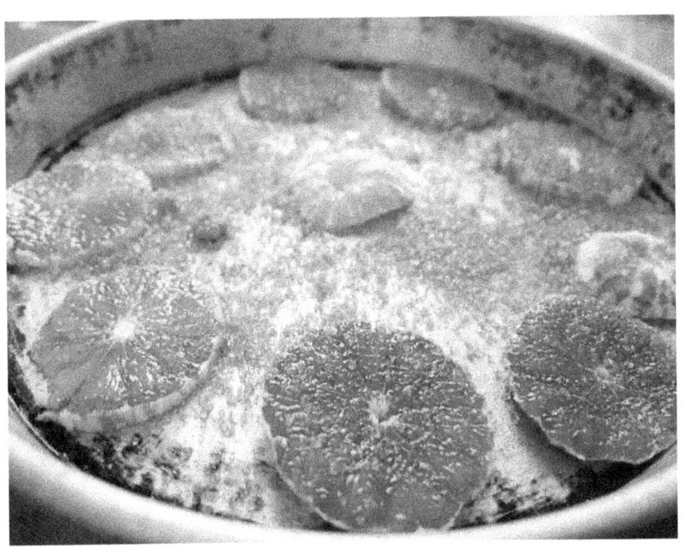

# Day 1

# Breakfast

**Eggs Scrambled Alongside Spinach and Tomatoes.**

Here's a recipe for delicious Scrambled Eggs with Spinach and Tomatoes:

**Ingredients:**

- 4 large eggs

- One cup of fresh baby spinach leaves, cut

- 1 medium tomato, diced

- 2 tablespoons milk (optional, for creamier eggs)

- Salt and pepper to taste

- 2 tablespoons cooking olive oil or butter

- Grated cheese (optional, for topping)

**Instructions:**

1. Prep the Ingredients:

- Wash the spinach leaves thoroughly and chop them into smaller pieces.

- Peel and dice the tomato into tiny pieces.

2. Whisk the Eggs:

- Break the eggs into a dish.

- Add milk if you want creamier eggs (this step is optional).

- Season with salt and pepper to taste.

- Whisk together the egg yolks and whites until fully mixed.

3. Heat the Pan:

- Melt butter in a nonstick skillet or frying pan at medium-low heat.

- Add the olive oil or butter and let it melt, ensuring it coats the bottom of the pan evenly.

4. Sauté the Vegetables:

- Add the diced tomatoes to the pan and sauté them for about 1-2 minutes until they start to soften.

5. Add Spinach:

- Add the chopped spinach to the pan with the tomatoes.

- Sauté for another 1-2 minutes, or until the spinach wilts and becomes tender.

6. Pour in the Eggs:

- Pour the beaten eggs into the pan with the sautéed spinach and tomatoes.

7. Scramble the Eggs:

- Using a spatula, gently stir the eggs and vegetables together.

- Keep stirring and folding the mixture over itself as the eggs begin to set.

8. Cook to Your Preferred Consistency:

- Continue cooking and stirring until the eggs reach your desired level of doneness. Some people prefer softer, moist scrambled eggs, while others like them fully cooked.

- Be careful not to overcook, as eggs can quickly become dry.

9. Season and Serve:

   - Season the scrambled eggs with a bit more salt and pepper if needed.

   - If desired, sprinkle some grated cheese on top of the eggs and let it melt.

10. Plate and Enjoy:

   - Transfer the scrambled eggs with spinach and tomatoes to a plate.

   - Serve hot, garnished with a little extra chopped spinach or diced tomato for freshness.

This simple and nutritious breakfast is packed with flavor and can be enjoyed on its own or with toast, a side of fruit, or your favorite breakfast accompaniments. Enjoy!

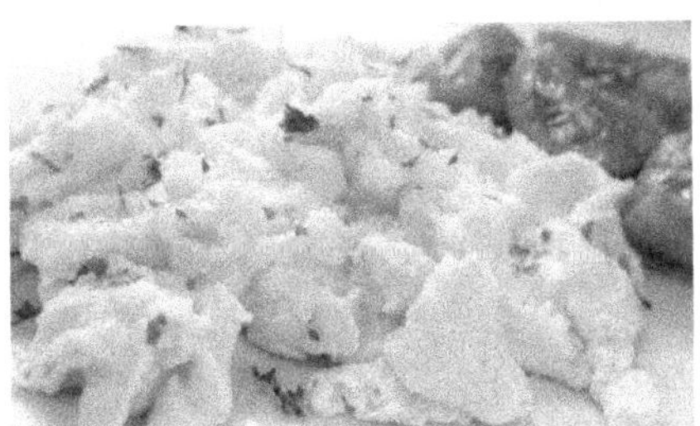

# Lunch

**Grilled Chicken Breast Salad with Mixed Greens, Cherry Tomatoes, Cucumbers, And A Vinaigrette Dressing.**

Here's a recipe for a delicious Grilled Chicken Breast Salad with Mixed Greens, Cherry Tomatoes, Cucumbers, and a Vinaigrette Dressing:

**Ingredients:**

**For the Salad:**

- 2 boneless, skinless chicken breasts

- Six cups mixed salad greens (e.g., lettuce, spinach, arugula)

- 1 cup cherry tomatoes, halved

- 1 cucumber, thinly sliced0

- 1/4 red onion, thinly sliced (optional)

- 1/4 cup crumbled feta cheese (optional)

- Salt and pepper to taste

- Olive oil for grilling

**For the Vinaigrette Dressing:**

- 3 tablespoons extra-virgin olive oil

- 1 tablespoon balsamic vinegar

- 1 teaspoon Dijon mustard

- 1 clove garlic, minced

- Salt and pepper to taste

**Instructions:**

**For the Grilled Chicken:**

1. Preheat the Grill:

   - Increase the temperature of your grill to medium-high.

2. Season the Chicken:

   - Sprinkle salt, pepper, and a little olive oil on the chicken breasts. You can also add your favorite herbs or spices for extra flavor.

3. Grill the Chicken:

- Place the chicken breasts on the preheated grill and cook for about 6-8 minutes per side, or until the chicken is no longer pink in the center and has nice grill marks.

- Cooking times may vary depending on the thickness of your chicken breasts, so you can use a meat thermometer to ensure they reach an internal temperature of 165°F (74°C).

4. Rest and Slice:

- Take the grilled chicken off the grill and give it some time to rest. Then, slice it into thin strips or cubes.

**For the Vinaigrette Dressing:**

1.Prepare the Dressing:

- Extra virgin olive oil, balsamic vinegar, Dijon mustard, minced garlic, salt, and pepper should all be incorporated into a small bowl. Taste the food and adjust the amount of seasoning as required.

Assemble the Salad:

1. Combine Ingredients:

- In a large salad bowl, combine the mixed salad greens, cherry tomatoes, sliced cucumber, and red onion (if using). Toss gently to mix.

2. Add Grilled Chicken:

- Arrange the sliced or cubed grilled chicken on top of the mixed greens.

3. Optional Toppings:

- If preferred, top the salad with crumbled feta cheese.

4. Drizzle with Dressing:

- Just before serving, drizzle the vinaigrette dressing over the salad.

5. Serve and Enjoy:

- Toss the salad to distribute the dressing throughout the entire dish.

- Serve immediately as a refreshing and satisfying meal.

This Grilled Chicken Breast Salad is a healthy and flavorful option, perfect for a light lunch or dinner. You can customize it with your favorite salad ingredients and adjust the dressing to your taste. Enjoy!

# Snack

**Greek Yogurt Dusted with Cinnamon.**

Greek yogurt with a sprinkle of cinnamon makes for a simple and healthy dessert or snack option. Here's how to prepare it:

**Ingredients:**

- 1 cup Greek yogurt (plain, non-fat, or low-fat)

- 1/2 teaspoon ground cinnamon

- If you want some sweetness, add some honey or maple syrup.

- Fresh fruit (optional, for garnish)

**Instructions:**

1. Prepare the Greek Yogurt:

  - Measure out 1 cup of Greek yogurt and place it in a serving bowl or dish.

2. Sprinkle with Cinnamon:

- Sprinkle the ground cinnamon evenly over the surface of the Greek yogurt. Use more or less cinnamon to suit your taste preferences.

3. Optional Sweetener:

- If you prefer your yogurt a bit sweeter, drizzle a small amount of honey or maple syrup over the yogurt. Start with a little and adjust to your desired level of sweetness.

4. Garnish with Fresh Fruit (Optional):

- For an extra burst of flavor and freshness, consider adding some fresh fruit on top. Sliced bananas, berries, or diced apples are all excellent choices. The fruit will complement the creamy yogurt and cinnamon beautifully.

5. Serve and Enjoy:

- Your Greek yogurt with a sprinkle of cinnamon is now ready to be enjoyed. Use a spoon to mix the cinnamon and sweetener (if used) into the yogurt before eating.

This quick and easy dessert is not only delicious but also packed with protein and calcium from Greek yogurt.

The cinnamon adds a warm and comforting flavor, making it a perfect treat for dinner or any time you want a healthy and satisfying dessert.

## Dinner

**Baked Salmon with Asparagus.**

Baked salmon with asparagus is a nutritious and flavorful dish that's easy to prepare. Here's a simple recipe for baked salmon with asparagus:

**Ingredients:**

- 2 salmon fillets (6-8 ounces each), skin-on or skinless, as preferred

- 1 bunch of fresh asparagus spears

- 2 tablespoons olive oil

- 2 cloves garlic, minced

- 1 lemon, thinly sliced

- Optional: one teaspoon of dill, either fresh or dried.

- To taste, add salt and freshly ground black pepper.

- Lemon wedges for garnish (optional)

- Dill or fresh parsley for garnish, if desired- Dill or fresh parsley for garnish, if desired

**Instructions:**

1. Preheat the Oven:

   - Set the oven's temperature to 375°F (190°C).

2. Prep the Asparagus:

   - Wash the asparagus spears and trim off the tough ends by snapping them off naturally at their breaking point.

3. Prepare the Salmon:

   - Place the salmon fillets on a clean cutting board or a plate. Pat them dry with paper towels.

   - Season both sides of the salmon with salt, freshly ground black pepper, and dried or fresh dill (if using). Set the seasoned salmon aside.

4. Prepare a Baking Sheet:

- For simpler cleanup, line a baking pan with parchment paper or aluminum foil.

- Drizzle 1 tablespoon of olive oil onto the lined baking sheet and spread it evenly.

5. Assemble the Dish:

- Place the salmon fillets, skin-side down if using skin-on fillets, on one side of the baking sheet.

- Arrange the asparagus spears on the other side of the baking sheet.

- Scatter the minced garlic evenly over the asparagus.

- Lay lemon slices on top of the salmon fillets and among the asparagus.

6. Drizzle with Olive Oil:

- Drizzle the remaining 1 tablespoon of olive oil over the salmon, asparagus, and lemon slices.

7. Bake in the Oven:

- Put the baking sheet in the hot oven, and bake it for 12 to 15 minutes. The thickness of your salmon fillets will determine the precise cooking time. The salmon is done when it flakes easily with a fork, and the asparagus is tender.

8. Serve:

- Remove the baking sheet from the oven with care.

- Garnish the dish with fresh parsley or dill and lemon wedges if desired.

9. Enjoy:

- Serve your baked salmon with asparagus immediately. The lemon-infused salmon and roasted asparagus create a delightful combination of flavors.

This baked salmon with asparagus recipe is not only delicious but also a healthy and well-balanced meal. It's ideal for a special event or a weeknight dinner.

# Day 2
# Breakfast

**Veggie Omelet:**

**Ingredients:**

- 2 large eggs

- 1/4 cup colored bell peppers, chopped

- 1/4 cup diced onions

- 1/4 cup diced mushrooms

- 1/4 cup diced tomatoes

- Salt and pepper to taste

- 1 teaspoon olive oil

- Optional: shredded cheese of your choice (for garnish)

**Instructions:**

1. In a nonstick skillet over moderately high heat, warm the olive oil.

2. In a bowl, beat the eggs and season with salt and pepper.

3. Pour the beaten eggs into the skillet, swirling to coat the bottom evenly.

4. Add the diced vegetables to one-half of the omelet.

5. Cook until the edges are set and the bottom is lightly browned.

6. Fold the omelet in half, covering the veggies.

7. If desired, sprinkle some shredded cheese on top.

8. Cook for another minute until the cheese melts.

9. Carefully slide the omelet onto a plate, cut it in half, and serve.

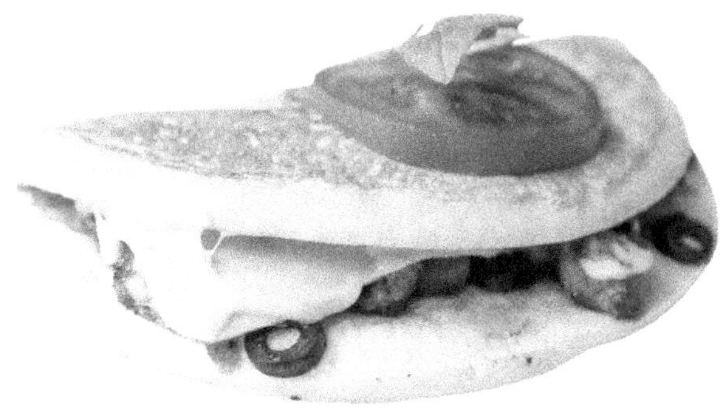

# Lunch

## Chicken Breast Packed with Spinach and Feta

### Ingredients:

- 2 boneless, skinless chicken breasts

- 1 cup fresh spinach leaves

- 1/4 cup crumbled feta cheese

- 2 cloves garlic, minced

- Salt and pepper to taste

- 1 tablespoon olive oil

- Toothpicks or kitchen twine for securing

### Instructions:

1. Preheat your oven to 375°F (190°C).

2. Butterfly each chicken breast by slicing horizontally, but not all the way through, to create a pocket.

3. Sprinkle salt and pepper inside the chicken breasts.

4. Stuff each chicken breast with spinach, feta cheese, and minced garlic.

5. Secure the openings with toothpicks or kitchen twine.

6. Heat olive oil in an ovenproof skillet over medium-high heat.

7. Sear the stuffed chicken breasts on both sides until golden brown.

8. Transfer the skillet to the preheated oven and bake for about 15-20 minutes or until the chicken is cooked through and no longer pink in the center.

9. Remove the toothpicks or twine before serving

# Snack

**Sliced Apple Ingredients:**

- 1 apple, thinly sliced

- 2 tbsp peanut butter (or almond butter)

**Instructions:**

1. Wash and thinly slice the apple.

2. Serve the apple slices with a small bowl of peanut butter for dipping.

3. Enjoy this simple and satisfying snack.

# Dinner

**Stir-Fried Tofu with Vegetables**

**Ingredients:**

-1 block of extra-firm tofu, cubed

- 2 cups mixed vegetables (e.g., broccoli, bell peppers, snap peas)

- 2 cloves garlic, minced

- 1 tablespoon ginger, minced

- 2 tablespoons low-sodium soy sauce

- 1 tablespoon hoisin sauce

- 1 tablespoon sesame oil

- 1 tablespoon vegetable oil

- Cooked quinoa or brown rice (for serving)

**Instructions:**

1.  In a big saucepan or wok, heat the vegetable oil on medium-high heat.
2.  2. Stir-fry the cubed tofu until it's lightly browned on all sides. Keep the tofu apart after removing it from the pan.
3.  In the same pan, add a bit more oil if needed, then add the minced garlic and ginger. Stir-fry for about 30 seconds.
4.  Stir-fry the mixed vegetables for 3-4 minutes, or until they begin to soften.
5.  Return the tofu to the pan and add the soy sauce, hoisin sauce, and sesame oil. Stir-fry for an additional 2-3 minutes to combine and heat everything through

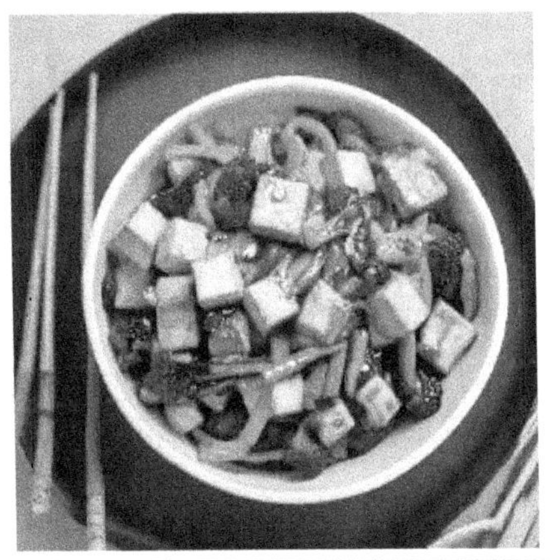

# Day 3

# Breakfast

**Greek Yogurt Parfait:**

**Ingredients:**

- 1 cup Greek yogurt (plain or flavored)
- 1/2 cup granola
- 1/2 cup mixed berries (e.g., strawberries, blueberries, raspberries)
- 1 tablespoon honey (optional, for drizzling)
- Chopped nuts (e.g., almonds or walnuts) for garnish (optional)

**Instructions:**

1. Begin with a layer of Greek yogurt in a glass or bowl.
2. Sprinkle granola on top of the yogurt.
3. Place a layer of mixed berries on top of the granola.
4. Repeat the layering until all of the ingredients have been utilized.
5. If desired, drizzle honey over the top for added sweetness.

6. Garnish with chopped nuts, if using.

7. Serve immediately and enjoy your delicious parfait!

# Lunch

**Lentil Soup**

**Ingredients:**

- 1 cup dried green or brown lentils
- 4 cups vegetable broth
- 1 onion, chopped
- 2 carrots, diced
- 2 celery stalks, diced
- 2 cloves garlic, minced
- 1 teaspoon cumin
- 1/2 teaspoon paprika
- Salt and pepper to taste
- Fresh parsley, chopped (for garnish)

**Instructions:**

1. In a large pot, heat a bit of olive oil over medium heat.

2. Add the chopped onion, carrots, celery, and garlic. Cook for 5 minutes, or until the vegetables soften.

3. Stir in the cumin and paprika.

4. Rinse the lentils under cold water and add them to the pot.

5. Pour in the vegetable broth.

6. Bring the mixture to a boil, then reduce the heat to a simmer and cover. Cook until the lentils are soft, about 20-25 minutes.

7. Season with salt and pepper to taste.

8. Garnish with fresh parsley before serving.

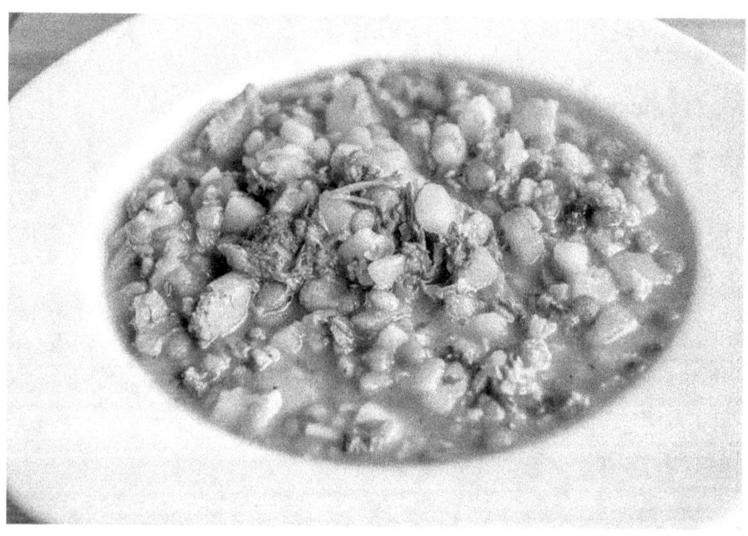

# Snack

**Veggie Sticks with Hummus**

**Ingredients:**

- Assorted fresh veggies (e.g., carrot sticks, cucumber slices, bell pepper strips, celery sticks)
- Hummus (store-bought or homemade)
- Optional: Cherry tomatoes or grape tomatoes for extra freshness

**Instructions:**

1. Wash and prepare the varied fresh veggies by cutting them into sticks, slices, or strips, depending on your preference.
2. Arrange the veggie sticks on a dish or serving tray.
3. Place a bowl of hummus in the center of the plate.
4. If desired, add some cherry tomatoes or grape tomatoes to the dish for more color and flavor.
5. Dip the veggie sticks into the hummus and enjoy this healthful and crispy snack.

6.  This snack is rich with vitamins, minerals, and fiber from the fresh vegetables, and the creamy hummus gives a delicious and delectable dip. It's a terrific technique to suppress hunger and enhance your energy in between meals.

# Dinner

**Grilled Lemon Herb Chicken with Quinoa And Roasted Vegetables**

**Ingredients:**

- For the Grilled Lemon Herb Chicken:
- 2 boneless, skinless chicken breasts
- 2 tablespoons olive oil
- 1 lemon, zested and juiced
- 2 cloves garlic, minced
- 1 teaspoon dried thyme
- 1 teaspoon dried rosemary
- Salt and pepper to taste

**For the Quinoa:**

- 1 cup quinoa

- 2 cups water or vegetable broth

- Salt to taste

**For the Roasted Vegetables:**

- Two cups of mixed vegetables (bell peppers, zucchini, cherry tomatoes, for example)

- 1 tablespoon olive oil

- Salt and pepper to taste

- Fresh basil leaves, for garnish (optional)

**Instructions:**

**For the Grilled Lemon Herb Chicken:**

1. In a bowl, whisk together olive oil, lemon zest, lemon juice, minced garlic, dried thyme, dried rosemary, salt, and pepper to create a marinade.

2. In a shallow dish or a resealable plastic bag, arrange the chicken breasts.

3. Coat the chicken completely with the marinade. Refrigerate or seal the bag for at least 30 minutes to allow the food to marinade.

4. Preheat your grill to medium-high heat.

5. Remove the chicken from the marinade and grill for about 6-8 minutes per side or until the chicken is cooked through and has grill marks.

6. Remove the chicken from the grill and allow it to rest for a few minutes before slicing.

## For the Quinoa:

1. Rinse the quinoa with cold water through a fine-mesh sieve.

2. In a saucepan, combine the cleaned quinoa and 2 cups of water or vegetable broth.

3. Season with salt to taste.

4. Bring the mixture to a boil, then decrease the heat to low, cover, and simmer for about 15-20 minutes or until the liquid is absorbed and the quinoa is fluffy.

5. Before serving, mix the quinoa with the tines of a fork.

## For the Roasted Vegetables

1. Preheat your oven to 400°F (200°C).

2. Toss the mixed vegetables with olive oil, salt, and pepper in a roasting pan or on a baking sheet.

3. In a preheated oven, roast the vegetables for 20-25 minutes, or until soft and slightly caramelized.

**To Serve:**

1. Divide the cooked quinoa among serving plates.
2. Top with sliced grilled lemon herb chicken.
3. Serve with roasted vegetables on the side.
4. Garnish with fresh basil leaves if preferred.
5. Enjoy your Grilled Lemon Herb Chicken with Quinoa and Roasted Vegetables!
6. This dinner is not only delicious but also balanced and nutritional, including lean protein, entire grains, and a variety of veggies for a full and wholesome meal.

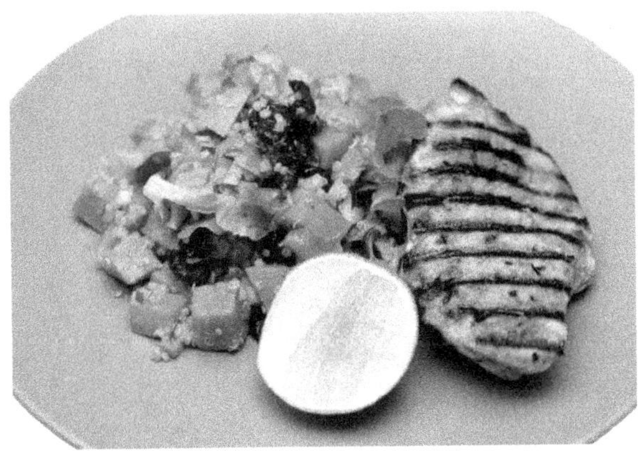

# Day 4

# Breakfast

**Avocado and Egg Breakfast Burrito**

**Ingredients:**

- 2 big eggs
- 1 large whole-grain tortilla
- 1/2 avocado, sliced
- 1/4 cup black beans, drained and rinsed
- 1/4 cup chopped tomatoes
- 2 tablespoons diced red onion
- 2 tablespoons shredded cheddar cheese
- Salt and pepper to taste
- Cooking spray or a tiny quantity of olive oil (for cooking)
- Remove from the skillet and set aside.

**Instructions:**

1. Scramble the Eggs:
- In a bowl, beat the eggs and season with salt and pepper to taste.

- Heat a non-stick skillet over medium heat and gently coat it with cooking spray or a small quantity of olive oil.
- Pour the beaten eggs into the skillet and heat, stirring regularly, until they are scrambled and cooked to your desired level of doneness. They should be taken out of the skillet and placed aside.

2. Assemble the Burrito:
- Lay the whole-grain tortilla on a clean surface.
- Place the sliced avocado in the center of the tortilla.
- Add the scrambled eggs, black beans, diced tomatoes, diced red onion, and shredded cheddar cheese on top of the avocado.

3. Fold and Roll:
- Carefully fold the sides of the tortilla inwards.
- Then, starting from the bottom, roll the tortilla tightly to make a burrito shape.

4. Optional: Warm the Burrito:
- If preferred, you can heat the completed burrito in a skillet for a few minutes on each side until it's warm and the cheese has melted.

**To Serve:**

- Place the Avocado and Egg Breakfast Burrito on a dish.
- You can chop it in half diagonally for easier eating.
- Enjoy your tasty and protein-packed breakfast burrito!
- This breakfast is not only tasty but also packed with healthy fats from the avocado, protein from the eggs and black beans, and fiber from the whole-grain tortilla. It's a fantastic way to start your day with energy and flavor.

# Lunch

**Chickpea and Quinoa Salad with Lemon-Tahini Dressing:**

**Ingredients:**

**For the Salad:**

- 1 cup cooked quinoa, cooled 1 can (15 oz.) clean and drained chickpeas
- 1 cup cucumber, diced 1 cup cherry tomatoes, halved 1/4 cup red onion, finely chopped 1/4 cup fresh parsley, chopped 1/4 cup fresh mint leaves, chopped (optional)
- Salt and pepper to taste

**For the Lemon-Tahini Dressing:**

- 3 tablespoons tahini
- Juice of 1 lemon
- 2 tablespoons olive oil
- 1 clove garlic, minced 2-3 tablespoons water (adjust for desired consistency)
- Salt and pepper to taste

**Instructions:**

**For the Salad:**

1. In a large bowl, add the cooked and cooled quinoa, chickpeas, sliced cucumber, halved cherry tomatoes, chopped red onion, fresh parsley, and fresh mint (if using).
2. Add a touch of pepper and salt according to your preferences when dressing the salad.

**For the Lemon-Tahini Dressing:**

1. In a small bowl, mix together tahini, lemon juice, olive oil, minced garlic, and water until smooth.

2. Add water gradually until you get your desired dressing consistency. If it's too thick, add a touch more water; if it's too thin, add more tahini.

3. Add a bit of pepper and salt according to your desire when creating the dressing.

**To Serve:**

- Drizzle the Lemon-Tahini Dressing over the salad.

- Toss everything together until the salad elements are equally coated with the dressing.

- Taste and adjust the seasoning if needed.

- Divide the Chickpea and Quinoa Salad into serving dishes.

- You can garnish with additional fresh herbs or a lemon wedge if desired.

- Enjoy your healthful and delightful lunch!

- This Chickpea and Quinoa Salad with Lemon-Tahini Dressing is a terrific alternative for a pleasant and healthful lunch. It's full of protein, fiber, and fresh vegetables, and the tangy tahini dressing gives a burst of flavor.

# Snack

**Hummus and Veggie Platter:**

**Ingredients:**

- 1/2 cup hummus (store-bought or homemade)
- Assorted fresh vegetables for dipping (e.g., carrot sticks, cucumber slices, bell pepper strips, cherry tomatoes, celery sticks)
- Olives (optional, for garnish)
- Fresh herbs like parsley or cilantro (optional, for garnish)

**Instructions:**

1. Wash and Prep Vegetables:
- Wash and prepare the varied fresh veggies by cutting them into sticks, slices, or strips, depending on your preference.
- Serve Hummus:
- Scoop the hummus into a serving bowl or platter, placing it in the center.

2.  Arrange Vegetables:

-   Surround the hummus with the varied fresh vegetables, putting them nicely on the plate.

-   Garnish (Optional):

-   If preferred, top the hummus with olives and fresh herbs like parsley or cilantro for extra flavor and presentation.

**Enjoy:**

-   Dip the fresh veggie sticks into the hummus and enjoy this nutritious and tasty snack.

-   This Hummus and veggie Platter is not only delicious but also rich with fiber, vitamins, and minerals from the vibrant array of vegetables. The creamy hummus creates a pleasant and tasty dip that works wonderfully with the crisp and crunchy veggies. It's a great option for a quick and nutritious snack.

# Dinner

**Baked Salmon with Garlic Butter and Roasted Vegetables**

**Ingredients:**

**For the Baked Salmon:**

- 2 salmon fillets (6-8 ounces each)
- 2 tablespoons melted butter
- 2 cloves garlic, minced 1 lemon, sliced
- Fresh dill (or your choice of fresh herbs)
- Salt and pepper to taste

**For the Roasted Vegetables:**

- 2 cups mixed vegetables (e.g., broccoli florets, bell peppers, zucchini, cherry tomatoes)
- 2 tablespoons olive oil
- Salt and pepper to taste

**Instruction**

1. For the Baked Salmon:
2. Set your oven's temperature to 375°F (190°C).

3.  The salmon fillets should be placed on a baking pan that has been lined with aluminum foil or parchment paper.

4.  Put some melted butter and minced garlic in a small bowl.

5.  The salmon fillets should be covered in the garlic butter mixture.

6.  Use salt and pepper to season the fish as you please.

7.  Each fillet should have lemon slices on top, along with fresh dill or any herbs of your choice.

8.  Bake for 12 to 15 minutes in the preheated oven, or until the salmon flakes easily and is evenly opaque.

9.  After removing the salmon from the oven, set it aside for a while before serving.

**Regarding the roasted veggies:**

-  Turn on the oven to 400 °F (200 °C). The mixed vegetables should be thoroughly coated in olive oil, salt, and pepper in a mixing bowl.

-  Place the vegetables in a single layer on a sheet of baking paper.

- Roast the vegetables for 20 to 25 minutes, stirring once halfway through, or until they are tender and barely caramelized.

**To Perform:**

- Put serving dishes with the baked salmon and garlic butter on them.
- Present next to the roasted vegetables.
- If desired, add additional fresh herbs as a garnish.
- Enjoy your delicious and healthy dinner!
- In addition to being delicious, this baked salmon with garlic butter and roasted vegetables is also loaded with protein, necessary fats, and a variety of vitamins and minerals from the vegetables. This dinner is balanced, simple to make, and ideal for a healthy evening.

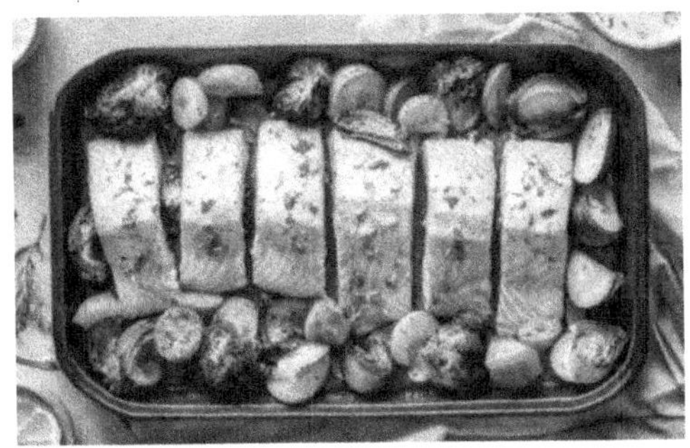

# Day 5

## Breakfast

**Oatmeal with mixed berries and almonds for breakfast:**

**Ingredients:**

- Oats, rolled, in a cup

- 1 cup milk, either dairy or vegan

- strawberries, blueberries, and raspberries make up half a cup of the mixed berries.

- 2tablespoons of almonds, sliced

- One spoonful of optionally flavor-enhancing honey or maple syrup

- a dash of cinnamon, if desired for flavor

**Instructions:**

1. Prepare the oats:

- In a saucepan, combine milk and rolled oats.

- If desired, add a dash of cinnamon for flavor.

- Bring the entire mixture to a simmer over medium-low heat.

- Stir and Simmer

- Oats should cook for around 5-7 minutes, stirring occasionally, or until they attain the desired level of thickness and creaminess.

2. Add almonds and berries:

- After taking the oats from the heat, stir in the chopped almonds and mixed berries.

- The oats' heat will gently soften the fruit.

3. Enhance (Optional):

- Add honey or maple syrup to your oats for added sweetness.

**To Serve:**

- Oatmeal should be transferred to a bowl

- If desired, garnish with additional berries, almonds, or a drizzle of honey.

- Enjoy your warm, filling breakfast of oats!

- A tasty and nutritious breakfast option is this oatmeal with mixed berries and almonds. The mixed berries give natural sweetness and antioxidants, and the oats offer fiber and sustained energy. It's a great way to start the day because the almonds provide a delicious crunch and beneficial lipids.

# Lunch

**Spinach and Feta Stuffed Chicken Breast for Lunch**

Heat the olive oil in an ovenproof skillet over medium-high heat.

**Ingredients:**

-   Regarding the Chicken Breast Stuffed:
-   2 skinless, boneless breasts of chicken
-   fresh spinach leaves, 1 cup
-   1/4 cup feta cheese crumbles
-   2 minced garlic cloves
-   pepper and salt as desired
-   (To be used in cooking)

**Relating to the lemon-herb quinoa:**

-   quinoa, one cup
-   2 cups of chicken broth or water
-   One lemon's juice and zest
-   one tablespoon of dried thyme
-   1 teaspoon of rosemary,
-   pepper and salt as desired

**Instructions:**

1. Regarding the Chicken Breast Stuffed:

2. Set your oven's temperature to 375°F (190°C).

3. Create a pocket in each chicken breast by cutting horizontally but not all the way through.

4. Salt and pepper the interior of the chicken breasts.

5. Each chicken breast should be stuffed with spinach, feta cheese, and minced garlic.

6. Use toothpicks or kitchen thread to close the gaps.

7. The olive oil should be heated in an ovenproof skillet over medium-high heat.

8. The stuffed chicken breasts should be cooked until golden brown on both sides.

9. When the chicken is cooked through and the middle is no longer pink, place the pan in the preheated oven and bake for about 15-20 minutes.

10. Before serving, take off the toothpicks or twine.

**Relating to the lemon-herb quinoa:**

- Using a fine-mesh strainer and cold water, rinse the quinoa.

- The cleaned quinoa, water or chicken broth, lemon zest, lemon juice, dried thyme, dried rosemary, salt, and pepper should all be combined in a pot.

- When the liquid is absorbed and the quinoa is fluffy, cook the mixture, covered, for 15 to 20 minutes after bringing it to a boil.

- Before serving, fluff the quinoa with a fork.

**To Perform:**

1. Place the Lemon Herb Quinoa next to the Spinach and Feta Stuffed Chicken Breast on the plate.

2. If you'd like, garnish with some fresh herbs or a wedge of lemon.

3. Enjoy your filling and enjoyable lunch!
   This lemon herb quinoa dish with spinach and feta filling is not only delicious, but it also has a good amount of protein, fiber, and other essential nutrients, making it a complete and well-balanced meal.

# Snack

**Greek yogurt and berry parfait for a snack**

**Ingredients:**

- 1 cup plain or vanilla-flavored Greek yogurt
- strawberries, blueberries, and raspberries make up half a cup of the mixed berries.
- 1/4 cup of cereal
- 1 tablespoon of optional, drizzle-able honey
- Nuts, such as almonds or walnuts, chopped for garnish

**Instructions:**

1. Adding Yog
2. In a glass or dish, start with an equal amount of Greek yogurt.
3. Insert the berries:
4. Mixed berries should be spread over the yogurt.
5. Add granola to the mixture:
6. Sprinkle granola over each of the berries.
7. Add a honey drizzle (optional):
8. If desired, drizzle honey on top for added sweetness.

9.  Add Nuts as a Garnish (Optional):

10. If you want to add a little crunch and extra protein, garnish with chopped nuts like almonds or walnuts.

**Serve right away:**

-   Enjoy this delicious and healthy Greek yogurt and berry parait as a snack!

In addition to being delicious, this parfait has a fantastic combination of protein from Greek yogurt, vitamins and fiber from the mixed berries, and a pleasant crunch from the granola and almonds. It's a great snack that will keep you satiated and energized all day.

# Dinner

**Vegetable Stir-Fry with Tofu and Brown Rice**

**Ingredients:**

**The stir-fry:**

-   1 cubed block of extra-firm tofu

-   2 cups of mixed veggies, such as carrots, bell peppers, snap peas, and broccoli florets

-   2 minced garlic cloves

- 1 teaspoon minced ginger

- Low-sodium soy sauce, 2 tablespoons

- A serving of hoisin sauce

- one teaspoon of sesame oil

- Vegetable oil, 1 tablespoon

- pepper and salt as desired

**Regarding the brown rice:**

- 1 serving brown rice

- 2-cups of water

- Salt as desired

**Instructions:**

The stir-fry

1. Making tofu:

- To press out extra moisture, press the tofu. It should be chopped up lightly seasoned and peppered.

2. Tofu stir-fry:

- Heat the vegetable oil over medium-high heat in a large skillet or wok.

The tofu should be stir-fried until it is gently browned all over. Remove the tofu from the pan and set it aside.

3.  Sauté ginger and garlic:
-   The minced garlic and ginger should be added to the same pan after a little extra oil if preferred. Stir-fry till fragrant after 30 seconds.
4.  Include Veggies:
-   The mixed vegetables should be added to the skillet and stir-fried for 3 to 4 minutes, or until they begin to soften.
5.  Sauces and Tofu Together:
-   Add the low-sodium soy sauce, hoisin sauce, and sesame oil to the pan with the tofu once more. Stir-fry for a further two to three minutes to completely combine and cook everything.

**Serve with seasoning:**

-   With salt and pepper, season the stir-fry to your taste.
-   Overcooked brown rice, plate the vegetable stir-fry.
-   Regarding the brown rice:

**Cleaning the Rice**

Brown rice should be soaked in cold water until transparent.

**Make rice:**

- Add water, a little salt, and the rinsed brown rice to a pot.
- Bring the mixture to a boil, then drop the heat to low, cover, and simmer for around 40-45 minutes or until the rice is cooked and the liquid is absorbed.
- With a fork, fluff the rice just before serving.

**To Perform:**

- Serve the brown rice separately when it has been cooked.
- Add the tofu mixture and vegetable stir-fry on top.
- If desired, garnish with sesame seeds or chopped green onions.
- Enjoy your delightful and wholesome Vegetable Stir-Fry with Tofu and Brown Rice!

This dinner is a full and delicious meal that includes protein-rich tofu, a variety of bright vegetables, and fiber-packed brown rice, all brought together with a savory stir-fry sauce. It's a good way to end the day with a nutritious and pleasurable meal.

# Day 6

## Breakfast

**Veggie and Cheese Omelette:**

**Ingredients:**

- 2 huge eggs
- 2 tablespoons milk (dairy or plant-based)
- pepper and salt as desired
- 1/4 cup sliced bell peppers (any color)
- 1/4 cup chopped tomatoes
- 1/4 cup diced onions
- 1/4 cup shredded cheddar cheese (or your favorite cheese)
- 1 teaspoon olive oil or butter (for cooking)
- Garnish with fresh herbs (e.g., parsley or chives) if liked.

**Instructions:**

1. Prepare the Veggies:
- In a small bowl, combine the diced bell peppers, diced tomatoes, and diced onions. These will be the filling for your omelet.

2. Whisk the Eggs:

- Whisk together the eggs and milk in a separate bowl until thoroughly combined.

- Season with salt and pepper according to desire.

3. Heat the Skillet:

- Heat a non-stick skillet over medium heat and add olive oil or butter. Make sure the oil or butter coats the bottom of the pan evenly.

4. Cook the Omelette:

- Fill the heated skillet with the whisked egg mixture.

- Allow the eggs to simmer for a minute or two, or until the edges begin to firm.

5. Add the Filling:

- Sprinkle the diced veggie mixture equally over one-half of the omelet.

- Add the shredded cheddar cheese on top of the veggies.

6. Fold and Finish:

- Carefully fold the other half of the omelet over the veggies and cheese, making a half-moon shape.

- Press down lightly with a spatula.

7. Cook Until Set:

- Continue cooking for another 2-3 minutes until the omelet is set but still somewhat runny on the inside.

**To Serve:**

- Slide the Veggie and Cheese Omelette onto a plate.
- Garnish with fresh herbs if desired.
- Enjoy your wonderful and protein-packed breakfast!
- This delicious Veggie and Cheese Omelette is the perfect way to kickstart your morning with a nutritious combination of protein from the eggs, vitamins, and fiber from the vegetables, and indulgent melted cheese. It's a fulfilling and wholesome breakfast choice.

# Lunch

**Caprese Salad Sandwich**

**Ingredients:**

- 2 servings of whole-grain bread (select bread with a low glycemic index)
- 2-3 pieces of raw mozzarella cheese
- 1 ripe tomato, thinly cut
- Fresh basil fronds

- 1 tablespoon extra-virgin olive oil

- 1 teaspoonful balsamic vinegar

- Salt and pepper to flavor

**Instructions:**

1. Prepare the Caprese Salad:

- In a bowl, combine the tomato slices, fresh basil leaves, and fresh mozzarella cheese segments.

2. Drizzle with Olive Oil and Balsamic Vinegar:

- Sprinkle the salad with extra-virgin olive oil and balsamic vinegar.

3. Season and Toss:

- To taste, season with a touch of salt and pepper.

- Gently mix the ingredients to coat them evenly with the dressing.

4. Assemble the Sandwich:

- Place one slice of whole-grain bread on a clear surface.

- Arrange the Caprese salad mélange on top of the bread.

5. Top with Second Slice:

- Place the second slice of whole-grain bread on top to create a sandwich.

**Serve:**

- Cut the Caprese Salad Sandwich in half diagonally if desired.
- Serve and appreciate your fresh and tasty lunch!

This light and refreshing Caprese Salad Sandwich has the classic blend of tomato, fresh mozzarella, and basil with a sprinkle of olive oil and balsamic vinegar. It's superb for a quick and nutritious meal.

# Snack

**Homemade Trail Mix**

**Ingredients**

- 1/2 cup unprocessed nuts (e.g., almonds, cashews, walnuts)
- 1/2 cup unprocessed seeds (e.g., pumpkin seeds, sunflower seeds)
- 1/2 cup dried fruits (raisins, cranberries, apricots, etc.)
- 1/4 cup dark chocolate pieces or chunks (optional)
- 1/4 cup whole-grain cereal (select a low glycemic index choice)

- 1/4 teaspoon salt (optional)

**Instructions:**

1. Select Your Ingredients:
- Choose a selection of nuts, seeds, and preserved fruits that you prefer. Ensure they are unsalted and free from additional sweeteners or oils.

2. Mix It Up:
- In a large bowl, combine the nuts, seeds, dried fruits, dark chocolate chunks (if using), and whole-grain cereal.
3. Add a Pinch of Salt (Optional):
- If you desire a trace of saltiness, you can add a pinch of salt to the mixture. However, this is optional and can be eliminated for a lower-sodium option.
4. Toss and Combine:
- Gently combine all the ingredients together until they are uniformly distributed.
5. Portion into Snack Bags:

- Divide the homemade trail mix into separate snack-sized packets or containers. This makes it simple to grab a bit when you need a fast snack.

6. Enjoy Your Custom Trail Mix:

- Whenever you're feeling hungry for a snack, take one of your pre-portioned packets of homemade trail mix.

It's a nutritious and enjoyable snack that delivers a combination of protein, healthy fats, fiber, and a hint of sweetness from the dried fruits and chocolate (if added).

This handmade trail mix allows you to personalize your refreshments to your preferences and dietary restrictions. It's a fantastic choice for on-the-go snacking and provides consistent energy throughout the day.

# Dinner

**Grilled Vegetable and Quinoa Stuffed Bell Peppers for Dinner**

**Ingredients:**

- For the Stuffed Bell Peppers:

- 4 enormous bell peppers (any color)

- 1 cup quinoa

- 2 cups water or vegetable bouillon

- 1 cup assorted grilled vegetables (e.g., zucchini, eggplant, red onion, cherry tomatoes)

- 1/2 cup feta cheese, shredded (optional)

- Fresh basil or parsley leaves, minced, for garnish (optional)

- Olive oil for scrubbing

- Salt and pepper to flavor

**For the Lemon-Herb Vinaigrette:**

- 2 tablespoons extra-virgin olive oil

- Juice of 1 lemon

- 1 clove garlic, minced

- 1 teaspoon dried thyme

- Salt and pepper to flavor

**Instructions:**

For the Stuffed Bell Peppers:

**Preheat the Grill:**

- Preheat your grill to medium-high heat.

## Prepare Quinoa:

- Rinse the quinoa under cool water using a fine-mesh sieve.
- In a saucepan, combine the rinsed quinoa and 2 cups of water or vegetable broth.
- Season with a sprinkle of salt.
- Bring the mixture to a boil, then decrease the heat to low, cover, and simmer for about 15-20 minutes or until the liquid is absorbed and the quinoa is frothy.
- Set aside the quinoa after fluffing it with a fork.

## Grill Vegetables:

- Brush the assorted vegetables (e.g., zucchini, eggplant, red onion, cherry tomatoes) with a little olive oil and season with salt and pepper.
- Grill the vegetables for 5-7 minutes, or until they are tender and have grill marks.
- Lift off the grill and chop into smaller segments.

## Prepare Bell Peppers:

- Remove the stems of the bell peppers and the seeds and membranes.
- Brush the outside of each bell pepper lightly with olive oil.
- Assemble Stuffed Peppers:
- In a large mixing basin, add the cooked quinoa and grilled vegetables.
- If preferable, add crumbled feta cheese for added taste.
- Stuff each bell pepper with the quinoa and veggie mixture, pressing it down slightly.

**Grill the Stuffed Peppers:**

- Place the stuffed bell peppers on the grill, cover, and cook for about 10-15 minutes, or until the peppers are faintly browned and soft.
- For the Lemon-Herb Vinaigrette:

**Prepare the Vinaigrette:**

- In a small basin, whisk together extra-virgin olive oil, lemon juice, minced garlic, dried oregano, salt, and pepper.

**To Serve:**

- Remove the loaded bell peppers from the grill and set them on serving plates.
- Drizzle the Lemon-Herb Vinaigrette over the top.
- If desired, top with fresh basil or parsley.

Enjoy your Grilled Vegetable and Quinoa Stuffed Bell Peppers! They're a delicious and nutritious dinner alternative.

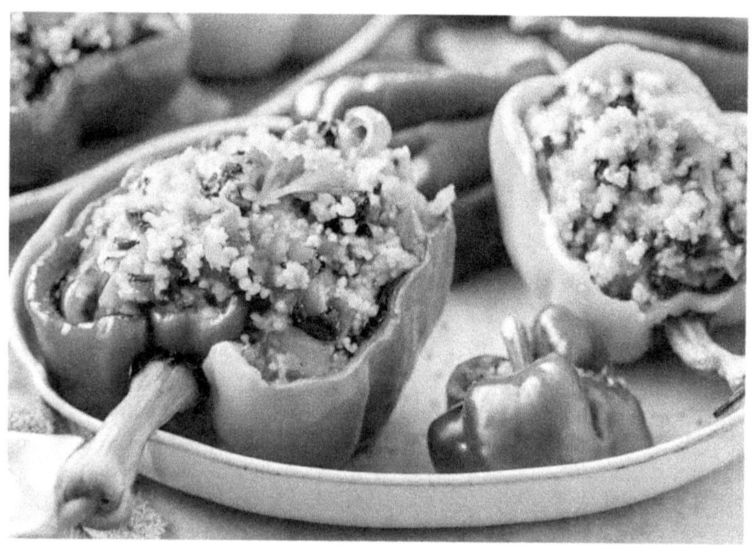

# Day 7

## Breakfast

**Berry and Almond Butter Overnight Oats:**

**Ingredients:**

- 1/2 cup rolled oats
- 1 cup milk (dairy or plant-based)
- 1/4 cup mixed berries (e.g., strawberries, blueberries, raspberries)
- 1 tablespoon almond butter (or your choice of nut butter)
- One tablespoon of honey or maple syrup (optional, for extra flavor)
- 1/4 teaspoon vanilla extract (optional)
- Sliced almonds for garnish (optional)

**Instructions:**

1.  Combine Ingredients:

-   In a mason jar or airtight container, combine the rolled oats, milk, mixed berries, almond butter, honey (or maple syrup), and vanilla extract (if using).

2.  Stir Well:

-   Stir in all of the ingredients until well incorporated.

3.  Refrigerate Overnight:

-   Chill the container overnight or for a minimum of 4 hours. The oats will absorb the liquid and become creamy as a result.

**Serve:**

-   When you're ready to eat, give the overnight oats a nice stir.

-   If the oats are too thick, you can add a bit more milk to attain your desired consistency.

Garnish (Optional):

-   Top with sliced almonds or extra berries for enhanced texture and flavor.

- Enjoy your convenient and nutritious breakfast!

These Berry and Almond Butter Overnight Oats are a terrific option for a hectic morning. They're packed with fiber, protein, and antioxidants from the berries, and the almond butter provides a creamy, nutty richness. Plus, it's a no-cook breakfast that's ready to go when you are! -

## Lunch

**Quinoa and Black Bean Salad with Avocado-Lime Dressing**

**Ingredients**

- For the Quinoa and Black Bean Salad:
- 1 cup cooked quinoa, cooled
- 1 can (15 oz) washed and drained black beans
- One cup of fresh, or canned corn kernels
- 1/2 cup red bell pepper, chopped
- 1/4 cup red onion, finely chopped
- 1/4 cup fresh cilantro, chopped (optional)
- Salt and pepper to taste

**For the Avocado-Lime Dressing:**

- 1 ripe avocado, peeled and pitted
- Juice of 2 limes
- 2 tablespoons extra-virgin olive oil
- 1 clove garlic, minced
- Salt and pepper to taste

**Instructions:**

**For the Quinoa and Black Bean Salad:**

1. Combine Ingredients:

In a large bowl, combine the cooked quinoa, black beans, corn kernels, sliced red bell pepper, minced red onion, and cilantro (if using).

2. Season:

Season the salad according to desire with salt and pepper.

**For the Avocado-Lime Dressing:**

1. Prepare the Dressing:

In a blender or food processor, combine the ripe avocado, lime juice, extra-virgin olive oil, minced garlic, salt, and pepper.

2. Blend Until Smooth:

Blend until the dressing is smooth and creamy. If it's too thick, you can add a bit of water to obtain your preferred consistency.

**To Serve:**

3. Drizzle Dressing:

Drizzle the Avocado-Lime Dressing over the Quinoa and Black Bean Salad.

4. Toss to Combine:

Toss everything together carefully until the salad is evenly coated in the dressing.

5. Garnish (Optional):

Garnish with more fresh cilantro or lime wedges if desired.

Enjoy your wonderful and nutritious lunch!

This Quinoa and Black Bean Salad with Avocado-Lime Dressing is not only tasty but also packed with protein, fiber, and healthy fats. It's a bright and vibrant salad that's excellent for a light and invigorating meal.

## Snack

**Veggie Sticks with Hummus:**

**Ingredients**

- Assorted fresh vegetable sticks (e.g., carrot sticks, cucumber slices, bell pepper strips, celery sticks)
- 1/2 cup hummus (store-bought or homemade)
- Cherry tomatoes and olives (optional, for garnish)
- Fresh herbs like parsley or cilantro (optional, for garnish)

**Instructions:**

1. Wash and Prep Vegetables:

Wash and prepare the varied fresh veggies by cutting them into sticks, slices, or strips, depending on your preference.

2. Serve Hummus:

Place the hummus in a serving bowl or on a plate.

3.  Arrange Veggie Sticks:

Surround the hummus with the varied fresh vegetable sticks, putting them nicely on the platter.

4.  Garnish (Optional):

If preferred, garnish the hummus with cherry tomatoes, olives, and fresh herbs like parsley or cilantro for extra flavor and presentation.

**Enjoy:**

Dip the fresh veggie sticks into the hummus and enjoy this nutritious and tasty snack.

Veggie Sticks with Hummus is a classic and nutritious snack choice. The fresh vegetables provide vitamins and minerals, while the hummus provides creaminess and protein, making it a fantastic alternative for a quick and healthy snack.

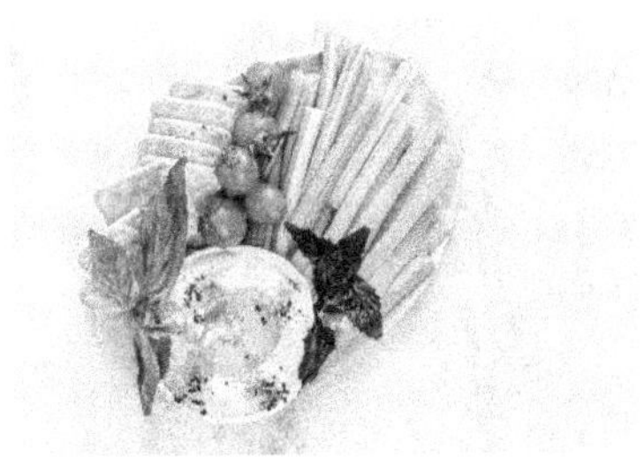

# Dinner

**Baked Chicken Breast with Roasted Vegetables:**

**Ingredients:**

- For the Baked Chicken Breast:
- 2 boneless, skinless chicken breasts
- 2 tablespoons olive oil
- 2 cloves garlic, minced
- 1 teaspoon dried thyme
- 1 teaspoon dried rosemary
- Salt and pepper to taste
- Lemon wedges for garnish (optional)

**For the Roasted Vegetables:**

- 2 cups mixed vegetables (e.g., broccoli florets, carrots, red bell peppers)
- 2 tablespoons olive oil
- Salt and pepper to taste

**Instructions:**

**For the Baked Chicken Breast:**

1. Preheat the Oven:

Preheat your oven to 375°F (190°C).

2. Season the Chicken:

Combine olive oil, minced garlic, dried thyme, dried rosemary, salt, and pepper in a small bowl.

3. Coat the Chicken:
- Place the chicken breasts on a baking sheet coated with parchment paper or in an ovenproof dish.
- Brush the chicken breasts with the herb and garlic mixture, ensuring they are coated evenly.

4. Bake the Chicken:

Bake for 25-30 minutes, or until the chicken is cooked through and no longer pink in the center, in a preheated oven. Internal temperature should be at 165°F (74°C).

5. Rest and Garnish:

- Remove the chicken from the oven and lay it aside for a few minutes to rest before slicing.

- Garnish with lemon wedges if preferred.

**For the Roasted Vegetables:**

6. Preheat the Oven:

While the chicken is baking, preheat your oven to 425°F (220°C).

7. Prepare Vegetables:

Toss the mixed veggies with olive oil, salt, and pepper in a mixing bowl until they are well-coated.

8. Roast the Vegetables:

On a baking sheet, put the seasoned vegetables in a single layer.

9. Roast in the Oven:

Roast the vegetables in a warm oven for 20-25 minutes, or until tender and slightly caramelized, stirring once halfway through.

**To Serve:**

- Place the sliced Baked Chicken Breast on serving plates.

- Serve alongside the Roasted Vegetables.

- Enjoy your wonderful and nutritious dinner!

This Baked Chicken Breast with Roasted Vegetables is a well-balanced dinner that's packed in protein, fiber, and vitamins from the vegetables. The herbs and garlic infuse the chicken with exquisite taste, and the roasted veggies offer a delectable side dish. It's a fantastic way to end your week with a nutritious and fulfilling dinner.

Remember to check your portion sizes, remain hydrated, and talk with a healthcare professional or a certified dietitian to modify this meal plan to your individual nutritional needs and blood sugar objectives. Additionally, be careful of your specific response to different foods and adapt the diet as needed.

# CHAPTER 5

## 50 extra Blood Sugar Recipes with Easy Prep Instruction and Time

## (Breakfast, Lunch, Dinner, Snacks, Disserts and Smoothies)

## Breakfast

## 1. Greek Yogurt Parfait:

**Ingredients:**

- 1 cup plain Greek yogurt (unsweetened)

- a half-cup of fresh berries (strawberries, blueberries, etc.)

- a quarter of a cup of chopped nuts (almonds, walnuts, etc.)

- 1 tablespoon honey (optional, for sweetness)

**Instructions:**

1. In a serving bowl or glass, start with a layer of Greek yogurt.

2. Add a layer of fresh berries.

3. Sprinkle chopped nuts on top.

4. Drizzle with honey if desired for added sweetness.

5. Repeat the layers if desired.

6. Serve as a protein-rich and satisfying breakfast.

Prep Time: 5 minutes

# 2. Vegetable Omelette:

**Ingredients:**

- 2 large eggs

- 1/4 cup diced bell peppers

- 1/4 cup diced tomatoes

- 1/4 cup diced onions

- 1/4 cup diced mushrooms

- 1 tablespoon olive oil

- Salt and pepper to taste

**Instructions:**

1. In a bowl, whisk together the eggs, salt, and pepper.

2. Heat olive oil in a non-stick skillet over medium-high heat.

3. Add diced bell peppers, tomatoes, onions, and mushrooms to the skillet. Sauté for about 2-3 minutes until they soften.

4. Pour the whisked eggs over the sautéed vegetables.

5. Cook until the edges start to set, then gently lift the edges to let the uncooked eggs flow to the edges.

6. Fold the omelet in half when it is mostly set but still somewhat runny on top.

7. Cook for another 1-2 minutes until it's fully cooked.

8. Serve hot as a protein-packed breakfast.

**Prep Time:** 10 minutes

# 3. Overnight Oats with Chia Seeds:

**Ingredients:**

- 1/2 cup rolled oats

- one cup of unsweetened almond milk (or your preferred milk)

- 1 tablespoon chia seeds

- 1/2 cup fresh berries (e.g., raspberries, blackberries)

- 1 tablespoon honey (optional, for sweetness)

**Instructions:**

1. In a jar or container, combine rolled oats, almond milk, and chia seeds.

2. Stir well to combine.

3. Top with a layer of fresh berries.

4. Drizzle with honey if desired for sweetness.

5. Cover the jar or container and refrigerate overnight.

6. In the morning, give it a good stir and enjoy your no-cook, fiber-rich breakfast.

**Prep Time:** 5 minutes (plus overnight refrigeration)

# 4. Spinach and Feta Breakfast Wrap:

**Ingredients:**

- 2 large eggs

- 1 cup fresh spinach leaves

- 2 tablespoons crumbled feta cheese

- 2 whole-grain or low-carb tortillas

- Olive oil for cooking

- Salt and pepper to taste

**Instructions:**

1. In a bowl, whisk together the eggs, salt, and pepper.

2. Heat a small non-stick skillet over medium-high heat with a little olive oil.

3. Add fresh spinach leaves to the skillet and sauté for about 1-2 minutes until they wilt.

4. Pour the whisked eggs over the wilted spinach.

5. Sprinkle crumbled feta cheese on top.

6. Cook until the eggs are set and the cheese is slightly melted.

7. Spread the tortillas out on a level surface.

8. Divide the egg and spinach mixture between the tortillas.

9. Roll the tortillas up, tucking the sides in as you go.

10. Serve as a protein-rich breakfast wrap.

**Prep Time:** 10 minutes

# 5. Almond and Berry Smoothie:

**Ingredients:**

- one cup of unsweetened almond milk (or your preferred milk)

- 1/2 cup fresh or frozen mixed berries (e.g., strawberries, blueberries)

- 1 tablespoon almond butter

- 1 tablespoon chia seeds

- 1/2 teaspoon ground cinnamon

- 1/2 teaspoon vanilla extract

- Ice cubes (optional)

**Instructions:**

1. In a blender, combine almond milk, mixed berries, almond butter, chia seeds, ground cinnamon, vanilla extract, and ice cubes if using.

2. Blend until smooth and creamy.

3. Pour into a glass and enjoy your nutritious and fiber-rich breakfast smoothie.

**Prep Time:** 5 minutes

# 6. Veggie and Cheese Breakfast Quesadilla:

**Ingredients:**

- 2 whole-grain or low-carb tortillas

- 2 large eggs, beaten

- 1/2 cup diced bell peppers

- 1/2 cup diced onions

- 1/2 cup shredded low-fat cheese

- Olive oil for cooking

- Salt and pepper to taste

**Instructions:**

1. Heat a small non-stick skillet over medium-high heat with a little olive oil.

2. Add diced bell peppers and onions to the skillet. Sauté for about 2-3 minutes until they soften.

3. Pour over the sautéed vegetables the beaten eggs.

4. Sprinkle shredded cheese on top.

5. Cook until the eggs are set and the cheese is melted.

6. Lay out the tortillas on a flat surface.

7. Divide the egg and vegetable mixture between the tortillas.

8. Roll the tortillas up, tucking the sides in as you go.

9. Serve as a protein-rich and satisfying breakfast quesadilla.

**Prep Time:** 10 minutes

# 7. Peanut Butter and Banana Overnight Oats

**Ingredients:**

- 1/2 cup rolled oats

- one cup of unsweetened almond milk (or your preferred milk)

- two tablespoons of natural peanut butter (no sugar added)

- 1 ripe banana, sliced

- 1/2 teaspoon ground cinnamon

- 1/2 teaspoon vanilla extract

- 1 teaspoon honey (optional, for sweetness)

**Instructions:**

1. In a jar or container, combine rolled oats, almond milk, peanut butter, sliced banana, ground cinnamon, vanilla extract, and honey if desired for sweetness.

2. Stir well to combine.

3. Refrigerate the jar or container overnight.

4. In the morning, give it a good stir, and enjoy your no-cook, protein-rich breakfast.

**Prep Time**: 5 minutes (plus overnight refrigeration)

# 8. Spinach and Mushroom Breakfast Burrito

**Ingredients:**

- 2 large eggs, beaten

- 1 cup fresh spinach leaves

- 1/2 cup sliced mushrooms

- 2 whole-grain or low-carb tortillas

- Olive oil for cooking

- Salt and pepper to taste

**Instructions:**

1. In a small non-stick skillet, heat a little olive oil over medium-high heat.

2. Add sliced mushrooms to the skillet and sauté for about 2-3 minutes until they soften.

3. Add fresh spinach leaves and sauté for another 1-2 minutes until they wilt.

4. Pour over the sautéed vegetables the beaten eggs.

5. Season with salt and pepper.

6. Cook until the eggs are set.

7. Spread the tortillas out on a level surface.

8. Divide the egg and vegetable mixture between the tortillas.

9. Roll the tortillas up, tucking the sides in as you go.

10. Serve as a protein-rich breakfast burrito.

**Prep Time:** 10 minutes

# 9. Cottage Cheese and Berries Bowl

**Ingredients:**

- 1 cup low-fat cottage cheese

- 1/2 cup fresh berries (e.g., raspberries, blueberries)

- 1 tablespoon chopped nuts (e.g., almonds, pecans)

- 1 teaspoon honey (optional, for sweetness)

**Instructions:**

1. In a serving bowl, place a layer of low-fat cottage cheese.

2. Top with fresh berries and chopped nuts.

3. Drizzle with honey if desired for added sweetness.

4. Serve as a protein-rich and satisfying breakfast bowl.

**Prep Time:** 5 minutes

# 10. Quinoa and Vegetable Breakfast Bowl (Vegetarian)

**Ingredients:**

- 1 cup cooked quinoa

- 1/2 cup diced bell peppers

- 1/2 cup diced tomatoes

- 1/4 cup diced red onion

- 1/4 cup crumbled feta cheese (optional)

- 1 tablespoon olive oil

- Salt and pepper to taste

- Fresh herbs (e.g., parsley, cilantro) for garnish

**Instructions**

1. In a bowl, combine cooked quinoa, diced bell peppers, diced tomatoes, diced red onion, and crumbled feta cheese (if using).

2. Drizzle with olive oil and season with salt and pepper.

3. Toss everything together gently.

4. Garnish with fresh herbs.

5. Serve as a fiber-rich and nutritious vegetarian breakfast bowl.

**Prep Time:** 15 minutes

These breakfast recipes offer a variety of flavors and ingredients to help you manage blood sugar levels while starting your day with a satisfying meal. They incorporate protein, fiber, and healthy fats for balanced nutrition. Adapt these recipes to your specific preferences and consult with a healthcare provider or registered dietitian for personalized guidance, especially if you have diabetes or other specific health concerns related to blood sugar management.

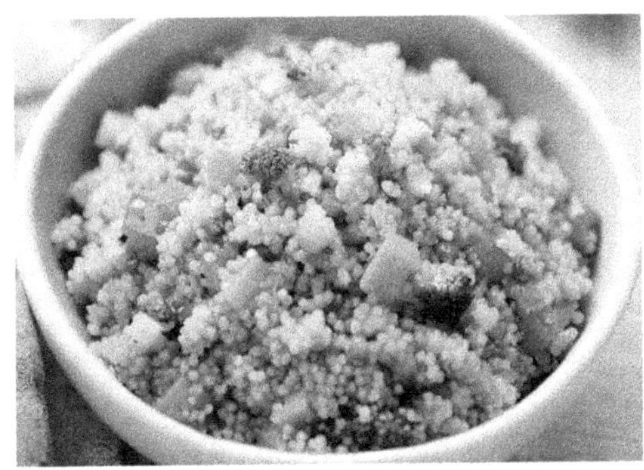

# Lunch

## 1. Chickpea and Avocado Salad

**Ingredients:**

- a single can (15 ounces) of washed and drained chickpeas

- 1 avocado, diced

- 1/2 cup cherry tomatoes, halved

- 1/4 red onion, finely chopped

- 1/4 cup fresh cilantro, chopped

- 2 tablespoons olive oil

- Juice of 1 lime

- Salt and pepper to taste

**Instructions:**

1. In a large bowl, combine chickpeas, diced avocado, cherry tomatoes, red onion, and fresh cilantro.

2. Drizzle with olive oil and lime juice.

3. Season according to preference with salt and pepper.

4. Toss everything together gently.

5. Serve as a refreshing and fiber-rich lunch.

**Prep Time:** 15 minutes

# 2. Turkey and Veggie Wrap

**Ingredients:**

- 4 whole-grain or low-carb tortillas

- 1/2-pound lean turkey breast, thinly sliced

- 1/2 cup hummus (low in added sugars)

- 1 cup mixed greens (e.g., spinach, arugula)

- 1/2 cucumber, thinly sliced

- 1/2 red bell pepper, thinly sliced

**Instructions:**

1. Spread the tortillas out on a flat surface.

2. Spread a layer of hummus onto each tortilla.

3. Add turkey slices, mixed greens, cucumber, and red bell
pepper.

4. Roll the tortillas up, tucking the sides in as you go.

5. Cut each wrap in half diagonally.

6. Serve as a satisfying and protein-packed lunch.

**Prep Time:** 15 minutes

# 3. Quinoa Salad with Roasted Vegetables (Vegetarian)

**Ingredients:**

- 1 cup quinoa

- 2 cups water or vegetable broth

- 2 cups roasted veggies (such as bell peppers, zucchini, and eggplant)

- 1/4 cup crumbled feta cheese (optional)

- 2 tablespoons olive oil

- 1 tablespoon balsamic vinegar

- Salt and pepper to taste

**Instructions:**

1. Rinse quinoa under cold water.

2. In a saucepan, combine quinoa and water or vegetable broth. Bring to a boil, then reduce heat, cover, and simmer for about 15-20 minutes until quinoa is cooked and liquid is absorbed.

3. While quinoa is cooking, toss mixed vegetables with olive oil, salt, and pepper. Roast in the oven at 400°F (200°C) for 15-20 minutes or until tender.

4. In a large bowl, combine cooked quinoa, roasted vegetables, and crumbled feta cheese (if using).

5. Toss with the balsamic vinegar to coat.

6. Serve as a hearty and nutritious vegetarian lunch.

**Prep Time:** 40 minutes

# 4. Tuna Salad Lettuce Wraps

**Ingredients:**

- 2 cans (5 ounces each) of tuna in water, drained

- 1/4 cup Greek yogurt (unsweetened)

- 1/4 cup diced celery

- 1/4 cup diced red onion

- 1 tablespoon lemon juice

- Salt and pepper to taste

- Large lettuce leaves (e.g., iceberg, Romaine)

**Instructions:**

1. In a bowl, combine drained tuna, Greek yogurt, diced celery, diced red onion, and lemon juice.

2. Season according to preference with salt and pepper.

3. Mix everything until well combined.

4. Spoon the tuna salad onto large lettuce leaves.

5. Roll up the leaves like wraps or tacos.

6. Serve as a low-carb and protein-rich lunch.

**Prep Time:** 15 minutes

# 5. Caprese Quinoa Bowl (Vegetarian)

**Ingredients:**

- 1 cup cooked quinoa

- 1 cup cherry tomatoes, halved

- 1 cup fresh mozzarella balls (mini)

- 1/4 cup fresh basil leaves

- 2 tablespoons balsamic glaze

- 1 tablespoon olive oil

- Salt and pepper to taste

**Instructions:**

1. In a bowl, combine cooked quinoa, cherry tomatoes, fresh mozzarella balls, and fresh basil leaves.

2. Drizzle with balsamic glaze and olive oil.

3. Season with salt and pepper to taste.

4. Toss everything together gently.

5. Serve as a light and flavorful vegetarian lunch.

**Prep Time:** 15 minutes

# 6. Spinach and Mushroom Quiche (Crustless, Vegetarian)

**Ingredients:**

- 4 large eggs

- 1 cup low-fat cottage cheese

- 1 cup fresh spinach, chopped

- 1 cup mushrooms, sliced

- 1/2 cup grated low-fat cheese (e.g., Swiss or mozzarella)

- 1/4 cup diced onion

- 1/4 teaspoon black pepper

- Olive oil for sautéing

**Instructions:**

1. Preheat your oven to 375°F (190°C).

2. In a skillet, sauté mushrooms and onions in olive oil until tender.

3. In a bowl, whisk together eggs, cottage cheese, chopped spinach, black pepper, and sautéed mushrooms and onions.

4. Pour the mixture into a pie plate that has been buttered.

5. Sprinkle grated cheese on top.

6. Bake for about 30-35 minutes until the quiche is set and lightly browned.

7. Allow it to cool for a few minutes before slicing.

8. Serve warm as a protein-packed vegetarian lunch.

Prep Time: 45 minutes

# 7. Shrimp and Avocado Salad:

**Ingredients:**

- a pound of large chopped and deveined shrimp

- 2 avocados, diced

- 1 cup cucumber, diced

- 1/4 cup red onion, finely chopped

- 1/4 cup fresh cilantro, chopped

- Juice of 2 limes

- 2 tablespoons olive oil

- Salt and pepper to taste

- Lettuce leaves (e.g., butter lettuce or Boston lettuce)

**Instructions:**

1. In a bowl, combine diced avocados, cucumber, red onion, and fresh cilantro.

2. Whisk together lime juice, olive oil, salt, and pepper in a separate bowl.

3. Season shrimp with salt and pepper.

4. Heat olive oil in a skillet over medium-high heat.

5. Add shrimp and cook for 2-3 minutes per side until they turn pink and opaque.

6. Toss the cooked shrimp with the dressing.

7. Arrange lettuce leaves on plates.

8. Top with the shrimp and avocado salad.

9. Serve as a light and refreshing lunch.

**Prep Time:** 30 minutes

# 8. Quinoa and Black Bean Bowl (Vegetarian)

**Ingredients:**

- 1 cup cooked quinoa

- a can (15 ounces) rinsed and drained black beans

1 cup corn kernels (fresh or frozen)

- 1/2 cup diced red bell pepper

- 1/4 cup chopped fresh cilantro

- 1/4 cup salsa (low in added sugars)

- Juice of 1 lime

- Salt and pepper to taste

- Sliced avocado (optional, for garnish)

**Instructions:**

1. In a large bowl, combine cooked quinoa, black beans, corn kernels, diced red bell pepper, and chopped cilantro.

2. In a separate small bowl, whisk together salsa, lime juice, salt, and pepper.

3. Toss the quinoa mixture with the dressing to combine it.

4. Garnish with sliced avocado if desired.

5. Serve as a flavorful and protein-rich vegetarian lunch.

**Prep Time:** 20 minutes

# 9. Grilled Vegetable and Chicken Wrap

**Ingredients:**

- 2 boneless, skinless chicken breasts

- 2 whole-grain or low-carb tortillas

- 1 cup mixed grilled vegetables (e.g., zucchini, eggplant, bell peppers)

- 2 tablespoons Greek yogurt (unsweetened)

- 1 tablespoon balsamic vinegar

- Salt and pepper to taste

**Instructions:**

1. Season chicken breasts with salt and pepper.

2. Grill the chicken for about 6-8 minutes per side until fully cooked.

3. Slice the grilled chicken into strips.

4. Spread the tortillas out on a level surface.

5. Spread a layer of Greek yogurt onto each tortilla.

6. Add sliced grilled chicken and mixed grilled vegetables.

7. Drizzle with balsamic vinegar.

8. Roll the tortillas up, tucking the sides in as you go.

9. Cut each wrap in half diagonally.

10. Serve as a protein-packed and satisfying lunch.

**Prep Time:** 30 minutes

# 10. Egg Salad Lettuce Wraps

Ingredients:

- 6 hard-boiled eggs, chopped

- 1/4 cup Greek yogurt (unsweetened)

- 1/4 cup diced celery

- 1/4 cup diced red onion

- 1 tablespoon Dijon mustard

- Salt and pepper to taste

- Big lettuce leaves (such as iceberg or Romaine)

**Instructions:**

1. In a bowl, combine chopped hard-boiled eggs, Greek yogurt, diced celery, diced red onion, Dijon mustard, salt, and pepper.

2. Mix everything until well combined.

3. Spoon the egg salad onto large lettuce leaves.

4. Roll up the leaves like wraps or tacos.

5. Serve as a protein-rich and low-carb lunch.

**Prep Time:** 20 minutes

These lunch recipes offer a variety of flavors and ingredients to help you manage blood sugar levels while enjoying a satisfying midday meal. They incorporate lean proteins, fiber-rich vegetables, and healthy fats for balanced nutrition. Adapt these recipes to your specific preferences and consult with a healthcare provider or registered dietitian for personalized guidance, especially if you have diabetes or other specific health concerns related to blood sugar management.

# Dinner

# 1. Baked Salmon with Asparagus:

**Ingredients:**

- 2 salmon fillets

- 1 bundle of asparagus spears

- 1 tablespoon olive oil

- Lemon slices

- Salt and pepper to taste

**Instructions:**

1. Preheat your oven to 375°F (190°C).

2. Place the salmon fillets on a baking pan lined with parchment paper.

3. Arrange asparagus spears around the salmon.

4. Drizzle olive oil over the salmon and asparagus, and season with salt and pepper.

5. Place lemon slices on top of the fish.

6. Bake for about 15-20 minutes, or until the salmon is cooked through and flakes easily with a fork.

7. Serve hot.

**Prep Time:** 25 minutes

# 2. Grilled Chicken Breast Salad:

**Ingredients:**

- 2 boneless, skinless chicken breasts

- 4 cups mixed greens (e.g., spinach, arugula, romaine)

- 1 cup cherry tomatoes, halved

- 1 cucumber, sliced

- 1/4 red onion, thinly sliced

- Olive oil and balsamic vinegar for dressing

- Salt and pepper to taste

**Instructions:**

1. Season the chicken breasts with salt and pepper.

2. Preheat a grill or grill pan over medium-high heat.

3. Grill the chicken for about 6-8 minutes per side, or until thoroughly done.

4. Slice the grilled chicken into strips.

5. In a large bowl, add mixed greens, cherry tomatoes, cucumber, and red onion.

6. Drizzle with olive oil and balsamic vinegar for dressing, and toss to coat.

7. Top the salad with cooked chicken strips.

8. Serve as a hearty and fulfilling meal.

**Prep Time:** 20 minutes

# 3. Quinoa and Vegetable Stir-Fry

**Ingredients:**

- 1 cup quinoa

- 2 cups water or veggie broth

- 2 tablespoons olive oil

- 1 bell pepper, thinly sliced

- 1 carrot, finely sliced

- 1 zucchini, thinly sliced

- 1 cup broccoli florets

- 2 cloves garlic, minced

- 2 tablespoons low-sodium soy sauce

- 1 tablespoon sesame oil

- Salt and pepper to taste

**Instructions:**

1. Rinse quinoa in cool water.

2. In a saucepan, add quinoa and water or vegetable broth. Bring to a boil, then reduce heat, cover, and simmer for about 15-20 minutes until quinoa is cooked and liquid is absorbed.

3. While quinoa is cooking, heat olive oil in a large skillet or wok over medium-high heat.

4. Add garlic, bell pepper, carrot, zucchini, and broccoli to the skillet. Stir-fry for around 5-7 minutes until the vegetables are tender-crisp.

5. Add cooked quinoa to the skillet and swirl to incorporate.

6. Drizzle with soy sauce and sesame oil, and season with salt and pepper.

7. Continue to cook for another 2-3 minutes.

8. Serve hot as a healthful and balanced supper.

**Prep Time:** 30 minutes

# 4. Lentil and Vegetable Soup

**Ingredients:**

- 1 cup dry green or brown lentils

- 4 cups vegetable broth

- 1 onion, chopped

- 2 carrots, chopped

- 2 celery stalks, chopped

- 2 cloves garlic, minced

- 1 teaspoon dried thyme

- 1 teaspoon dried rosemary

- Salt and pepper to taste

**Instructions:**

1. Rinse lentils with cool water.

2. In a large soup pot, heat a dab of olive oil over medium heat.

3. Add chopped onion, carrots, celery, and garlic. Sauté for around 5 minutes until the vegetables soften.

4. Add lentils, vegetable broth, dried thyme, dried rosemary, salt, and pepper to the pot.

5. Bring to a boil, then reduce heat, cover, and simmer for about 20-25 minutes until the lentils are cooked.

6. Serve hot as a hearty and fiber-rich meal.

**Prep Time:** 40 minutes

# 5. Stuffed Bell Peppers

**Ingredients**

- 4 bell peppers (any color)

- 1 cup cooked quinoa or brown rice

- 1 cup lean ground turkey or lean ground beef

- 1 cup chopped tomatoes (canned or fresh)

- 1/2 cup black beans (canned, drained, and rinsed)

- 1/2 cup maize kernels (fresh or frozen)

- 1 teaspoon chili powder

- 1/2 teaspoon cumin

- Salt and pepper to taste

- Shredded low-fat cheese (optional, for topping)

**Instructions:**

1. Preheat your oven to 375°F (190°C).

2. Cut the tops off the bell peppers and remove the seeds and membranes.

3. In a skillet, brown the ground turkey or beef over medium heat. Drain any extra fat.

4. Add chopped tomatoes, black beans, corn, chili powder, cumin, salt, and pepper to the skillet. Cook for an additional 5 minutes.

5. Stir in the cooked quinoa or brown rice.

6. Fill each bell pepper with the meat and quinoa mixture.

7. Place the stuffed bell peppers in a baking dish and cover with aluminum foil.

8. Bake for about 25-30 minutes until the peppers are cooked.

9. Optionally, put shredded low-fat cheese on top during the last 5 minutes of baking.

10. Serve hot as a tasty and balanced meal.

**Prep Time**: 50 minutes

# 6. Zucchini Noodles with Pesto and Cherry Tomatoes

**Ingredients:**

- 2 large zucchinis (spiralized into noodles)

- Olive oil for sautéing

- Salt and pepper to taste

Instructions:

1. Heat olive oil in a large skillet over medium-high heat.

2. Add zucchini noodles and sauté for 2-3 minutes until slightly tender

3. Stir in cherry tomatoes and simmer for an additional 2 minutes.

4. Remove from heat and stir with basil pesto.

5. Sprinkle with Parmesan cheese if desired.

6. Serve immediately.

**Prep Time:** 15 minutes

# 7. Baked Chicken Thighs with Roasted Vegetables

**Ingredients:**

- 4 bone-in, skin-on chicken thighs

- 2 cups mixed vegetables (e.g., bell peppers, broccoli, cauliflower)

- 2 tablespoons olive oil

- 1 teaspoon dry herbs (e.g., thyme, rosemary)

- Salt and pepper to taste

**Instructions:**

1. Preheat your oven to 375°F (190°C).

2. Season chicken thighs with dried herbs, salt, and pepper.

3. Arrange chicken and mixed vegetables on a baking sheet.

4. Drizzle olive oil over everything.

5. Bake for about 35-40 minutes or until chicken is cooked through and vegetables are soft.

6. Serve hot.

**Prep Time:** 45 minutes

# 8. Lentil and Vegetable Stir-Fry (Vegetarian)

**Ingredients:**

- 1 cup green or brown lentils

- 2 cups water or veggie broth

- 2 tablespoons olive oil

- 1 bell pepper, thinly sliced

- 1 carrot, finely sliced

- 1 zucchini, thinly sliced

- 1 cup broccoli florets

- 2 cloves garlic, minced

- 2 tablespoons low-sodium soy sauce

- 1 tablespoon sesame oil

- Salt and pepper to taste

**Instructions:**

1. Rinse lentils with cool water.

2. In a saucepan, add lentils and water or vegetable broth. Bring to a boil, then decrease heat, cover, and simmer for about 15-20 minutes until lentils are cooked and liquid is absorbed.

3. While lentils are cooking, heat olive oil in a large skillet or wok over medium-high heat.

4. Stir in the garlic, bell pepper, carrot, zucchini, and broccoli. Cook for 5-7 minutes, or until the vegetables are tender-crisp.

5. Add cooked lentils to the skillet and swirl to mix.

6. Drizzle with soy sauce

7. Continue to cook for another 2-3 minutes.

8. Serve hot as a healthful and balanced vegetarian supper.

Prep Time: 40 minutes

# 9. Baked Cod with Spinach and Tomatoes

**Ingredients:**

- 4 cod fillets

- 2 cups fresh spinach

- 1 cup cherry tomatoes, halved

- 2 cloves garlic, minced

- 1 lemon (zested and juiced)

- 2 tablespoons olive oil

- Salt and pepper to taste

**Instructions:**

1. Preheat your oven to 375°F (190°C).

2. In a large oven-safe skillet, heat olive oil over medium-high heat.

3. Add minced garlic and sauté for about 1 minute until fragrant.

4. Stir in the fresh spinach and cherry tomatoes. Cook for about 2-3 minutes or until the spinach wilts.

5. Season cod fillets with salt, pepper, and lemon zest. Place them on top of the spinach and tomatoes.

6. Drizzle with lemon juice.

7. Transfer the skillet to the oven and bake for 15-20 minutes or until the fish is cooked through and flakes easily with a fork.

8. Serve hot.

**Prep Time:** 30 minutes

# 10. Shrimp and Broccoli Stir-Fry

**Ingredients:**

About a pound of big peeled and deveined shrimp

- 2 cups broccoli florets

- 1 red bell pepper, thinly sliced

- 2 cloves garlic, minced

- 2 tablespoons low-sodium soy sauce

- 1 tablespoon hoisin sauce

- 1 teaspoon sesame oil

- 1 teaspoon grated ginger

- Olive oil for stir-frying

- Salt and pepper to taste

**Instructions:**

1. In a bowl, whisk together low-sodium soy sauce, hoisin sauce, sesame oil, grated ginger, and a touch of salt and pepper.

2. Heat olive oil in a large skillet or wok over medium-high heat.

3. Add minced garlic and stir-fry for about 1 minute until fragrant.

4. Cook for 2-3 minutes, or until the shrimp turn pink. Take away after pulling out of the skillet.

5. In the same skillet, add a bit extra olive oil if needed. Stir-fry broccoli and red bell pepper for around 4-5 minutes until tender-crisp.

6. Return the cooked shrimp to the skillet and pour the sauce over everything

7. Stir-fry for another 2 minutes until the shrimp are heated through and coated in the sauce.

8. Serve hot.

**Prep Time:** 25 minutes

These supper dishes offer a range of flavors and ingredients to help you regulate blood sugar levels while having a great meal. They combine lean proteins, fiber-rich vegetables, and healthy fats for balanced nourishment. As always, individual dietary needs may vary, so it's essential to adapt these recipes to your specific preferences and consult with a healthcare provider or registered dietitian for personalized guidance, especially if you have diabetes or other specific health concerns related to blood sugar management.

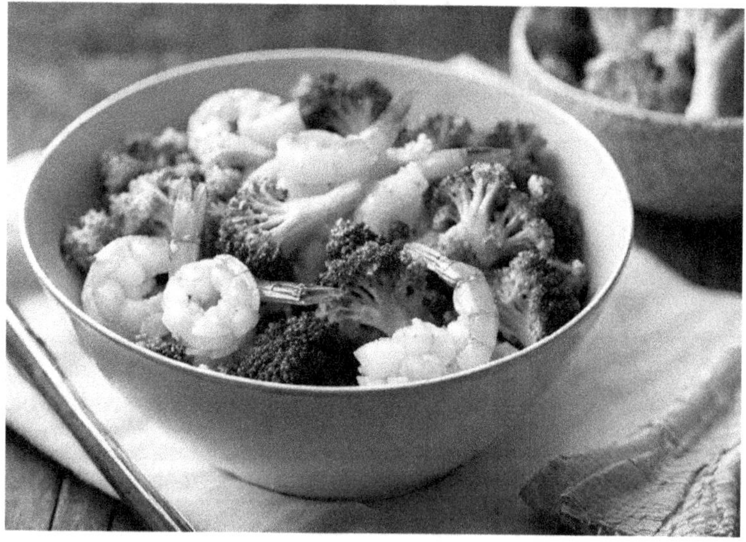

# Snacks

# 1. Greek Yogurt and Berries Parfait

**Ingredients:**

- 1 cup Greek yogurt (unsweetened)

- half a cup of berries (strawberries, blueberries, raspberries, etc.)

- 1 tablespoon chopped nuts (e.g., almonds, walnuts)

- 1 teaspoon honey (optional)

**Instructions:**

1. In a glass or bowl, layer Greek yogurt, mixed berries, and chopped nuts.

2. Drizzle with honey for added sweetness if desired.

3. Serve immediately.

**Prep Time:** 5 minutes

# 2. Cucumber and Hummus Slices

**Ingredients:**

- 1 cucumber

- 1/4 cup hummus (low in added sugars)

- Cherry tomatoes (optional, for garnish)

**Instructions:**

1. Slice the cucumber into rounds or sticks.

2. Serve with a side of hummus for dipping.

3. Garnish with cherry tomatoes if desired.

Prep Time: 5 minutes

# 3. Cottage Cheese with Sliced Peaches

**Ingredients:**

- 1/2 cup low-fat cottage cheese

- 1 ripe peach, sliced

- 1/2 teaspoon cinnamon (optional)

Instructions:

1. Place the cottage cheese in a mixing basin.

2. Top with sliced peaches.

3. Sprinkle with cinnamon for extra flavor if desired.

**Prep Time**: 5 minutes

# 4. Veggie Sticks with Guacamole

**Ingredients:**

- Assorted fresh vegetable sticks (e.g., carrot sticks, cucumber slices, bell pepper strips)

- 1 ripe avocado

- 1/2 lime (juiced)

- 1 clove garlic (minced)

- Salt and pepper to taste

**Instructions:**

1. Prepare the vegetable sticks.

2. In a bowl, mash the ripe avocado.

3. Stir in lime juice, minced garlic, salt, and pepper to make guacamole.

4. Serve the vegetable sticks with guacamole for dipping.

**Prep Time:** 10 minutes

# 5. Almonds and Cheese

**Ingredients:**

- 1/4 cup unsalted almonds

- 1 small piece of cheese (e.g., string cheese, cheddar, or Swiss)

**Instructions:**

1. Measure out the almonds.

2. Pair with a small piece of cheese.

3. Enjoy a balanced and filling snack.

**Prep Time:** 2 minutes

# 6. Sliced Apples with Almond Butter

**Ingredients**

- 1 apple (sliced)

- 2 tablespoons almond butter (unsweetened)

**Instructions:**

1. Slice the apple.

2. Serve with almond butter for dipping or spreading.

3. A sprinkle of cinnamon can be added for extra flavor.

**Prep Time:** 5 minutes

# 7. Hard-Boiled Eggs

**Ingredients:**

- 2 hard-boiled eggs

- Salt and pepper to taste

**Instructions:**

1. Prepare hard-boiled eggs in advance.

2. Sprinkle with a pinch of salt and pepper.

3. Enjoy a protein-rich snack.

**Prep Time:** 10 minutes (includes boiling time)

# 8. Edamame Snack:

**Ingredients:**

- 1 cup edamame (cooked and shelled)

- A pinch of sea salt

**Instructions:**

1. Steam or boil the edamame until tender.

2. Sprinkle with a pinch of sea salt.

3. Serve as a nutritious and protein-packed snack.

**Prep Time:** 5 minutes

# 9. Rice Cakes with Avocado

**Ingredients:**

- 2 rice cakes (choose low glycemic index)

- 1 ripe avocado

- Cherry tomatoes (optional, for garnish)

**Instructions:**

1. Spread mashed avocado onto rice cakes.

2. Garnish with cherry tomatoes if desired.

3. Serve as a crunchy and creamy snack.

**Prep Time:** 5 minutes

# 10. Tomato and Mozzarella Caprese Skewers

**Ingredients:**

- Cherry tomatoes

- Fresh mozzarella balls (mini)

- Fresh basil leaves

- Balsamic vinegar (optional, for drizzling)

**Instructions:**

1. Thread cherry tomatoes, mozzarella balls, and basil leaves onto skewers.

2. Drizzle with balsamic vinegar for added flavor if desired.

3. Enjoy as a refreshing and savory snack.

**Prep Time:** 10 minutes

These snack recipes are designed to be lower in added sugars and incorporate ingredients that are generally lower on the glycemic index to help manage blood sugar levels. They also provide a balance of nutrients, including fiber, protein, and healthy fats.

However, individual responses to foods can vary, so it's essential to monitor your blood sugar levels and adjust recipes to meet your specific dietary needs and preferences. Additionally, it's advisable to consult with a healthcare provider or registered dietitian for personalized dietary guidance, especially if you have diabetes or other specific health concerns related to blood sugar management.

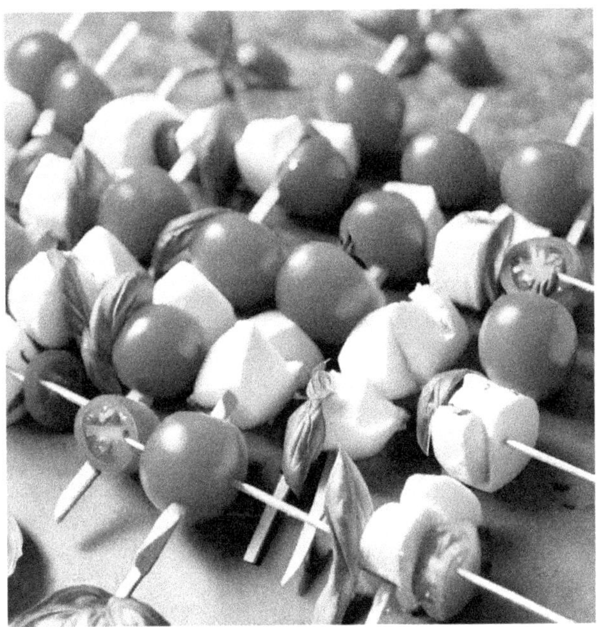

# Desserts

## 1. Berry Parfait

**Ingredients:**

- 1 cup Greek yogurt (unsweetened)

- a half-cup of mixed berries (blueberries, raspberries, etc.)

- 1 tablespoon chopped nuts (e.g., almonds, walnuts)

- 1 teaspoon honey (optional)

**Instructions:**

1. In a glass or bowl, layer Greek yogurt, mixed berries, and chopped nuts.

2. Drizzle with honey for added sweetness if desired.

3. Serve immediately.

**Prep Time:** 5 minutes

## 2. Baked Apples with Cinnamon

**Ingredients:**

- 2 apples

- 1 teaspoon cinnamon

- 1 tablespoon chopped walnuts (optional)

**Instructions:**

1. Preheat the oven to 350°F (175°C).

2. Peel and core the apples, then set them in a baking pan.

3. Sprinkle cinnamon over the apples and add chopped walnuts.

4. Bake for about 25-30 minutes until apples are tender.

5. Serve warm.

**Prep Time:** 35 minutes

# 3. Chia Seed Pudding

**Ingredients:**

- 3 tablespoons chia seeds

- 1 cup unsweetened almond milk

- 1/2 teaspoon vanilla extract

- Fresh berries for topping

**Instructions:**

1. In a bowl, combine chia seeds, almond milk, and vanilla extract.

2. Stir well and refrigerate overnight.

3. Top with fresh berries before serving.

**Prep Time:** 5 minutes (plus overnight chilling)

# 4. Chocolate Avocado Mousse

**Ingredients:**

- 2 ripe avocados

- 1/4 cup unsweetened cocoa powder

- 2-3 tablespoons honey or a sugar substitute

- 1 teaspoon vanilla extract

**Instructions:**

1. Blend avocados, cocoa powder, honey (or sugar substitute), and vanilla extract until smooth.

2. Place in the refrigerator for at least 30 minutes before serving.

3. Garnish with berries if desired.

**Prep Time:** 10 minutes

# 5. Greek Yogurt with Almond Butter and Berries

**Ingredients:**

- 1 cup Greek yogurt (unsweetened)

- 2 tablespoons almond butter

- 1/2 cup mixed berries

**Instructions:**

1. In a bowl, combine Greek yogurt and almond butter.

2. Top with mixed berries.

3. Drizzle with honey for added sweetness if desired.

**Prep Time:** 5 minutes

# 6. Cinnamon-Spiced Baked Pears

**Ingredients:**

- 2 ripe pears

- 1/2 teaspoon cinnamon

- 1 tablespoon chopped pecans (optional)

**Instructions:**

1. Preheat the oven to 375°F (190°C).

2. Cut pears in half and remove the cores.

3. Sprinkle cinnamon and chopped pecans over the pears.

4. Bake for about 20-25 minutes until pears are tender.

5. Serve warm.

**Prep Time:** 30 minutes

# 7. Mixed Berry Sorbet

**Ingredients:**

- 2 cups mixed berries (e.g., strawberries, blueberries, raspberries)

- 1 tablespoon lemon juice

- 1-2 tablespoons honey or a sugar substitute

**Instructions:**

1. Blend mixed berries, lemon juice, and honey (or sugar substitute) until smooth.

2. Pour into an ice cream machine and churn according to package directions.

3. Serve immediately as soft-serve or freeze for a firmer texture.

**Prep Time:** 10 minutes (plus freezing time)

# 8. Almond and Coconut Energy Bites

**Ingredients:**

- 1 cup rolled oats

- 1/2 cup almond butter

- 1/4 cup shredded coconut (unsweetened)

- 1/4 cup chopped almonds

- 1/4 cup ground flaxseed

A quarter cup of honey (or a sugar alternative)

- 1 teaspoon vanilla extract

**Instructions:**

1. In a bowl, combine all ingredients.

2. Roll the mixture into bite-sized balls.

3. Place in the refrigerator for about 30 minutes before serving.

**Prep Time:** 15 minutes

# 9. Mini Cheesecakes with Berry Topping

**Ingredients:**

- 1 cup low-fat cream cheese

- 1/4 cup Greek yogurt (unsweetened)

A quarter cup of honey (or a sugar alternative)

- 1 egg

- 1 teaspoon vanilla extract

- 1/2 cup mixed berries for topping

**Instructions:**

1. Preheat the oven to 325°F (160°C).

2. In a bowl, beat together cream cheese, Greek yogurt, honey (or sugar substitute), egg, and vanilla extract until smooth.

3. Pour the mixture into mini muffin tins.

4. Bake for about 15-18 minutes until set.

5. Let them cool and top with mixed berries.

**Prep Time:** 25 minutes

# 10. Pumpkin Chia Pudding:

**Ingredients:**

- 1/2 cup canned pumpkin puree

- 2 tablespoons chia seeds

- 1/2 cup unsweetened almond milk

- 1/2 teaspoon pumpkin pie spice

- 1-2 tablespoons honey or a sugar substitute (adjust to taste)

**Instructions:**

1. In a bowl, mix pumpkin

 puree, chia seeds, almond milk, pumpkin pie spice, and honey (or sugar substitute).

2. Chill for a minimum of a two-hour period or overnight.

3. Serve chilled, garnished with a sprinkle of cinnamon.

Prep Time: 5 minutes (plus chilling time)

These dessert recipes are designed to be lower in added sugars and incorporate ingredients that are generally lower on the glycemic index to help manage blood sugar levels. However, individual responses to foods can vary, so it's essential to monitor your blood sugar levels and adjust recipes to meet your specific dietary needs and preferences. Additionally, it's advisable to consult with a healthcare provider or registered dietitian for personalized dietary guidance, especially if you have diabetes or other specific health concerns related to blood sugar management.

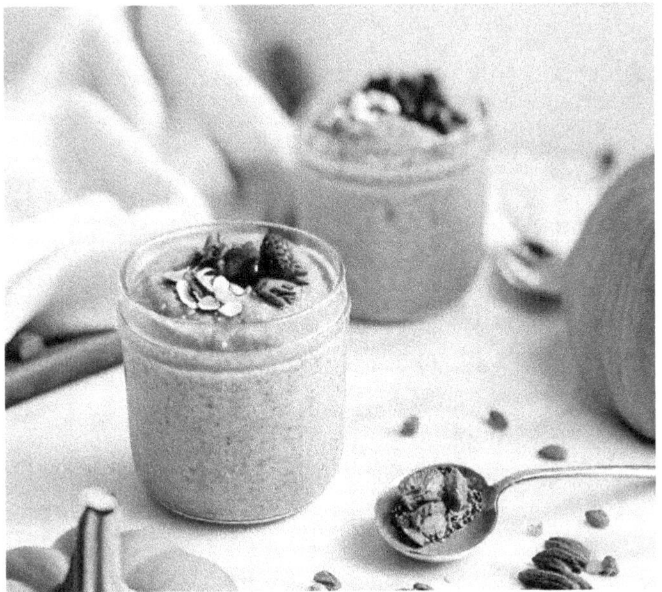

# Smoothies

## 1. Green Power Smoothie:

**Ingredients:**

- 1 cup spinach (fresh or frozen)

- 1/2 medium avocado

- 1/2 cucumber

- 1/2 green apple (cored and peeled)

- 1/2 cup unsweetened almond milk

- 1 tablespoon chia seeds (optional)

- Ice cubes (optional)

**Instructions:**

1. Place spinach, avocado, cucumber, green apple, and almond milk in a blender.

2. Blend until smooth.

3. Add chia seeds and ice cubes (if desired) and blend again.

4. Serve immediately.

# 2. Berry and Greek Yogurt Smoothie

**Ingredients:**

- 1/2 cup Greek yogurt (unsweetened)

- half a cup of berries (strawberries, blueberries, raspberries, etc.)

- 1 tablespoon ground flaxseed

- 1/2 teaspoon cinnamon

- half a cup of unscented almond milk or water

- Ice cubes (optional)

**Instructions:**

1. Combine Greek yogurt, mixed berries, ground flaxseed, cinnamon, and water (or almond milk) in a blender.

2. Blend until smooth.

3. Add ice cubes if you prefer a colder texture and blend again.

4. Serve immediately.

**Prep Time:** 5 minutes

# 3. Tropical Turmeric Smoothie

**Ingredients:**

- 1/2 cup frozen pineapple chunks

- 1/2 cup frozen mango chunks

- 1/2 teaspoon turmeric powder

- 1/2 teaspoon ginger (fresh or ground)

- 1 tablespoon chia seeds

- 1 cup unsweetened coconut milk (or water)

- Ice cubes (optional)

**Instructions:**

1. Combine frozen pineapple, mango, turmeric, ginger, chia seeds, and coconut milk (or water) in a blender.

2. Blend until smooth.

3. Add ice cubes if you'd like a colder consistency and blend again.

4. Serve immediately.

**Prep Time:** 5 minutes

# 4. Cinnamon and Banana Smoothie

**Ingredients:**

- 1 ripe banana

- 1/2 teaspoon cinnamon

- 1 tablespoon almond butter

- 1/2 cup unsweetened almond milk

- 1/4 cup Greek yogurt (unsweetened)

- Ice cubes (optional)

**Instructions:**

1. Blend the ripe banana, cinnamon, almond butter, almond milk, and Greek yogurt until smooth.

2. Add ice cubes if you prefer a colder texture and blend again.

3. Serve immediately.

**Prep Time:** 5 minutes

# 5. Blueberry and Almond Smoothie:

**Ingredients:**

- 1/2 cup frozen blueberries

- 1/4 cup unsalted almonds

- 1 tablespoon almond butter

- 1/2 teaspoon vanilla extract

- 1 cup unsweetened almond milk

- Ice cubes (optional)

**Instructions:**

1. Blend frozen blueberries, unsalted almonds, almond butter, vanilla extract, and almond milk until smooth.

2. Add ice cubes if you want a colder consistency and blend again.

3. Serve immediately.

**Prep Time:** 5 minutes

# 6. Spinach and Banana Protein Smoothie

**Ingredients:**

- 1 cup spinach (fresh or frozen)

- 1 ripe banana

- 1 scoop of unflavored or vanilla protein powder (low in sugar)

- 1/2 cup unsweetened almond milk

- 1/2 cup water

- Ice cubes (optional)

**Instructions:**

1. Combine spinach, ripe banana, protein powder, almond milk, and water in a blender.

2. Blend until smooth.

3. Add ice cubes if you want a colder texture and blend again.

4. Serve immediately.

**Prep Time:** 5 minutes

# 7. Peanut Butter and Cocoa Smoothie:

**Ingredients:**

- 1 tablespoon peanut butter (unsweetened)

- 1 tablespoon cocoa powder (unsweetened)

- 1/2 ripe banana

- 1/2 cup unsweetened almond milk

- 1/2 cup Greek yogurt (unsweetened)

- Ice cubes (optional)

**Instructions:**

1. Blend peanut butter, cocoa powder, ripe banana, almond milk, and Greek yogurt until smooth.

2. Add ice cubes if you'd like a colder consistency and blend again.

3. Serve immediately.

**Prep Time:** 5 minutes

# 8. Chia and Mixed Berry Protein Smoothie

**Ingredients:**

- half a cup of berries (strawberries, blueberries, raspberries, etc.)

- 1 tablespoon chia seeds

- 1 scoop unflavored

 or vanilla protein powder (low in sugar)

- 1/2 cup unsweetened almond milk

- 1/2 cup water

- Ice cubes (optional)

**Instructions:**

1. Blend mixed berries, chia seeds, protein powder, almond milk, and water until smooth.

2. Add ice cubes if you want a colder texture and blend again.

3. Serve immediately.

**Prep Time**: 5 minutes

# 9. Pumpkin Spice Smoothie

**Ingredients:**

- 1/2 cup canned pumpkin puree (unsweetened)

- 1/2 teaspoon pumpkin pie spice

- 1 tablespoon almond butter

- 1/2 cup unsweetened almond milk

- 1/2 cup Greek yogurt (unsweetened)

- Ice cubes (optional)

**Instructions:**

1. Blend pumpkin puree, pumpkin pie spice, almond butter, almond milk, and Greek yogurt until smooth.

2. Add ice cubes if you'd like a colder consistency and blend again.

3. Serve immediately.

**Prep Time:** 5 minutes

# 10. Kiwi and Kale Green Smoothie

**Ingredients:**

- 1 kiwi (peeled and sliced)

- 1 cup kale leaves (stems removed)

- 1/2 banana

- 1/2 cup unsweetened almond milk

- 1/2 cup water

- Ice cubes (optional)

**Instructions:**

1. Blend kiwi, kale leaves, banana, almond milk, and water until smooth.

2. Add ice cubes if you want a colder texture and blend again.

3. Serve immediately.

**Prep Time:** 5 minutes

These smoothie recipes are designed to be lower in added sugars and incorporate ingredients that are generally lower on the glycemic index to help manage blood sugar levels. They also provide a balance of nutrients, including fiber, healthy fats, and protein. However, individual responses to foods can vary, so it's essential to monitor your blood sugar levels and adjust recipes to meet your specific dietary needs and preferences. Additionally, it's advisable to consult with a healthcare provider or registered dietitian for personalized dietary guidance, especially if you have diabetes or other specific health concerns related to blood sugar management.

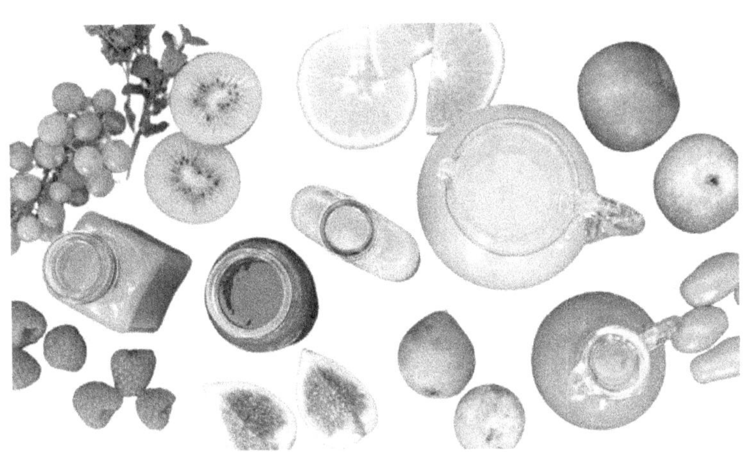

# CHAPTER 6

## Exercise and Physical Activity

Exercise has a major impact on blood sugar levels and can play a critical role in blood sugar management, particularly for persons with diabetes or those at risk of developing the condition.

The relationship between exercise and blood sugar is complex and multifaceted. Here's how exercise affects blood sugar:

1. Improved Insulin Sensitivity:

Regular physical activity boosts insulin sensitivity, helping the body's cells to better respond to insulin's messages. When you exercise, your muscles use glucose for energy, minimizing the requirement for insulin to enhance glucose uptake. This enhanced sensitivity helps reduce blood sugar levels.

2. Immediate Glucose Utilization:

During exercise, muscles require extra glucose for energy.

To meet this need, the body accelerates the uptake of glucose from the bloodstream into muscle cells, leading to a transient dip in blood sugar levels.

This impact can be particularly advantageous for persons with diabetes to prevent post-meal increases.

3. Reduced Insulin Resistance:

Exercise can lower insulin resistance, a hallmark of type 2 diabetes. It does so by stimulating the migration of glucose transporters (GLUT-4) to the cell surface, making it easier for cells to take up glucose in response to insulin.

4. Improved Glycemic Control:

Engaging in regular physical activity can lead to better overall glycemic management, which involves maintaining stable blood sugar levels throughout the day. It helps avoid both hyperglycemia (high blood sugar) and hypoglycemia (low blood sugar) episodes.

5. Weight Management:

Exercise can aid with weight management, which is vital for blood sugar regulation.

Maintaining a healthy weight minimizes insulin resistance and enhances the body's capacity to manage blood sugar.

6. Enhanced Muscle Glucose Storage:

Exercise stimulates the accumulation of glucose in muscle tissue in the form of glycogen. This stored glucose might be utilized during repeated bouts of physical exercise or when blood sugar levels dip.

7. Improved Post-Meal Blood Sugar:

Engaging in physical activity after a meal can help minimize post-meal blood sugar rises. A brisk stroll or modest exercise can boost glucose uptake by muscle cells, minimizing the requirement for extra insulin.

8. Long-Term Benefits:

Consistent exercise over time can lead to enduring improvements in blood sugar control. Regular physical exercise correlates to better HbA1c (average blood sugar levels over several months) and minimizes the risk of problems linked with poorly managed blood sugar.

9. Stress Reduction:

Exercise can help reduce stress, which can have a favorable impact on blood sugar levels. High-stress levels can lead to high cortisol levels, which, in turn, can contribute to insulin resistance.

10. Individual Variability:

It's crucial to note that the impact of exercise on blood sugar levels can differ from person to person. Factors such as the type, length, and intensity of exercise, as well as an individual's fitness level, medication use, and food, all have a part in determining how exercise affects blood sugar.

11. Monitoring and Adjustments:

Individuals with diabetes should monitor their blood sugar levels before, during, and after exercise to learn how their body responds. Depending on the reaction, modifications may be needed in terms of food consumption, insulin or medication doses, and the timing and intensity of exercise.

In conclusion, exercise has a dramatic impact on blood sugar levels and plays a critical role in blood sugar regulation.

Regular physical activity can enhance insulin sensitivity, promote glucose use by muscles, and contribute to better overall glycemic management. It is a crucial component of a holistic approach to diabetes care and can contribute to long-term health and well-being. Individuals with diabetes should engage with healthcare providers to design an activity regimen tailored to their unique requirements and goals.

# Creating an Effective Exercise Routine (10 exercises that Impact blood sugar)

let's empathize and list 10 exercises that affect blood sugar levels and specify their impact:

**1. Brisk Walking:**

Description: Imagine taking a vigorous stroll in your neighborhood. Your pulse rate is elevated, and you're breaking a light sweat.

Impact: Brisk walking is like a mild nudge to your blood sugar. It helps your muscles utilize glucose for energy, leading to a quick decline in blood sugar levels. Over time, regular walks improve insulin sensitivity and maintain stable blood sugar control.

## 2. Jogging:

Description: Picture yourself jogging in a local park, setting a steady speed that's faster than walking.

Impact: Jogging is like a slow decline in your blood sugar levels. It burns calories, promotes glucose uptake by muscles, and enhances insulin sensitivity. It's helpful for long-term blood sugar regulation and weight control.

## 3. Cycling:

Description: Imagine cycling along a gorgeous trail. Your legs push the pedals, and the wind rushes by you.

Impact: Cycling is a dynamic workout that might have an immediate influence on blood sugar. It burns carbs for energy, resulting in lowered blood sugar levels during and after the ride. Over time, it promotes insulin sensitivity and supports weight management.

## 4. Swimming:

Description: Visualize yourself swimming laps in a pool. The water offers resistance as you move your arms and legs.

Impact: Swimming is a full-body workout that can drop blood sugar levels while you're in the pool. The water's buoyancy decreases the impact on your joints, making it a good option for persons with joint concerns. Over time, it adds to greater insulin sensitivity.

## 5. Resistance Training:

Description: Picture yourself lifting weights or utilizing resistance bands at the gym. Your muscles contract against resistance.

Impact: Resistance training improves your muscles, which can lead to increased glucose uptake. As your muscles grow more effective at utilizing glucose, blood sugar levels tend to stabilize. It also helps with weight management and long-term blood sugar control.

## 6. Yoga:

Description: Imagine a tranquil yoga session, when you glide through mild positions and focus on your breath.

Impact: While yoga may not have an immediate impact on blood sugar, it helps alleviate stress. Lower stress levels can indirectly assist better blood sugar control by reducing cortisol, a hormone that can influence insulin sensitivity.

## 7. High-Intensity Interval Training (HIIT):

Description: Picture yourself doing short bursts of vigorous workouts like sprinting or jumping jacks, followed by brief periods of rest.

Impact: HIIT workouts provide a punch for blood sugar. They contribute to quick glucose utilization and an immediate decline in blood sugar levels. Over time, HIIT can considerably improve insulin sensitivity and enhance overall cardiovascular fitness.

## 8. Dancing:

Description: Visualize dancing to your favorite song. Your body moves rhythmically, and you're having pleasure.

Impact: Dancing is not only pleasurable but also an excellent way to lower blood sugar levels. It combines aerobic and muscle-strengthening activities, boosting glucose uptake and enhancing insulin sensitivity.

## 9. Pilates:

Description: Imagine practicing Pilates, focusing on core strength and flexibility exercises.

Impact: Pilates may not contribute to immediate changes in blood sugar, but it increases muscle tone and strength. Over time, it helps to better glucose management and supports overall fitness.

## 10. Tai Chi:

Description: Picture yourself doing Tai Chi in a quiet park. You move fluidly through a sequence of flowing, slow-motion positions.

Impact: Tai Chi helps relieve stress and improve balance and flexibility. While it may not have an immediate influence on blood sugar, it can indirectly assist better blood sugar control by lowering stress levels.

Remember, the influence of exercise on blood sugar might vary from person to person, and consistency is crucial. Choose activities you enjoy and can sustain over time, and consider working with a healthcare professional or a fitness expert to personalize your workout regimen to your unique needs and goals. Exercise, combined with a balanced diet and other healthy lifestyle choices, can greatly improve blood sugar management and general well-being.

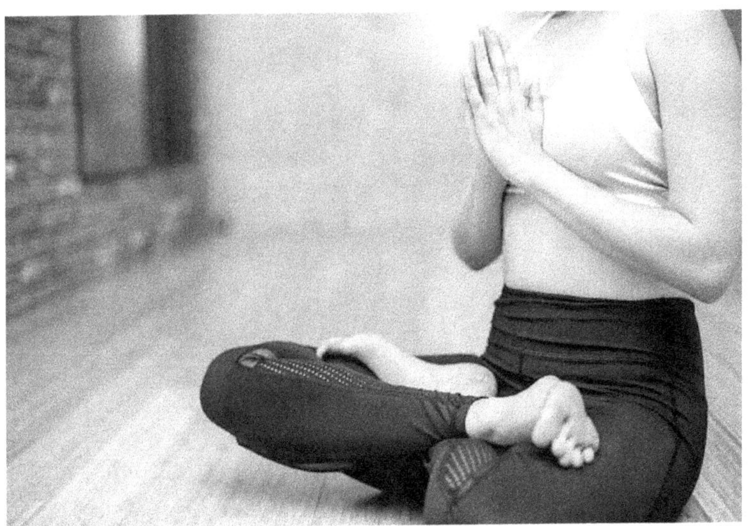

# Stress Management and Sleep

Stress management and sleep play pivotal roles in blood sugar management. The connection between these factors is intricate, and mastering techniques for stress reduction and achieving quality sleep can significantly impact your blood sugar control. In this comprehensive guide, we will delve into the relationship between stress, sleep, and blood sugar and explore effective techniques to address these aspects of diabetes management.

The Relationship between Stress, Sleep, and Blood glucose:

1. Stress and Blood Sugar: Stress triggers the release of hormones, including cortisol and adrenaline, which can lead to increased blood sugar levels. This response, often referred to as the "fight or flight" reaction, provides the body with extra energy in stressful situations. However, chronic stress can result in consistently elevated blood sugar, making it challenging to manage diabetes effectively.

2. Stress and Food Choices: Stress can influence food choices, leading to cravings for sugary or high-carbohydrate foods.

These comfort foods may provide momentary relief from stress but can result in blood sugar spikes, exacerbating diabetes management difficulties.

3. Sleep and Blood Sugar: Inadequate or poor-quality sleep can disrupt the body's ability to regulate blood sugar. Sleep deprivation can lead to insulin resistance, causing blood sugar levels to rise. Additionally, irregular sleep patterns can affect circadian rhythms, further impacting glucose control.

4. Sleep and Appetite Regulation: Sleep plays a critical role in appetite regulation. Insufficient sleep can disrupt hormones that control hunger and fullness, potentially leading to overeating and unhealthy food choices, which can, in turn, affect blood sugar levels.

# Techniques for Stress Reduction and Quality Sleep:

1. Mindfulness Meditation: Practicing mindfulness meditation involves staying present in the moment, focusing on your breath, and letting go of stressors. Regular mindfulness meditation can reduce stress and improve sleep quality.

2. Deep Breathing Exercises: Deep breathing techniques, such as diaphragmatic breathing and progressive muscle relaxation, help calm the nervous system, reduce stress, and prepare the body for restful sleep.

3. Physical Activity: Regular exercise, such as walking, swimming, or yoga, can reduce stress and promote better sleep. Engaging in physical activity earlier in the day can also aid in falling asleep more easily at night.

4. Stress Management Techniques: Explore stress management techniques like journaling, art therapy, or engaging in hobbies you enjoy. These activities can serve as effective outlets for stress.

5. Establish a Relaxing Bedtime Routine: Create a calming bedtime routine that signals to your body that it's time to wind down. This may include reading, taking a warm bath, or practicing gentle stretches.

6. Limit Screen Time: Reduce exposure to screens (phones, computers, TVs) before bedtime, as the blue light emitted from screens can interfere with sleep by disrupting melatonin production.

7. Keep a Consistent Sleep Schedule: Sleep and wake up at the same times every day, including on weekends. This helps to adjust your body's internal clock and increase the quality of your sleep.

8. Create a Sleep-Friendly Environment: Make your bedroom conducive to sleep by keeping it cool, dark, and quiet. Invest in a comfortable mattress and pillows that support restful sleep.

9. Limit Caffeine and Alcohol Intake: Reduce caffeine consumption in the afternoon and evening, as it can interfere with sleep. Similarly, limit alcohol consumption, which can disrupt sleep patterns.

10. Seek Professional Help: If stress or sleep disturbances persist, consider seeking support from a mental health professional or sleep specialist. They can provide targeted strategies and interventions to address your specific concerns.

11. Blood Sugar Monitoring: Regularly monitor your blood sugar levels, especially during periods of increased stress or when sleep quality is compromised. This helps you proactively manage any fluctuations.

In conclusion, stress management and quality sleep are integral components of effective blood sugar management. The connection between stress, sleep, and blood sugar levels underscores the importance of addressing these aspects of your health. By incorporating stress reduction techniques and adopting sleep-enhancing practices into your daily routine, you can significantly improve your blood sugar control, overall well-being, and quality of life. Remember that achieving better blood sugar management is a holistic journey that involves not only monitoring your glucose levels but also nurturing your emotional and physical health.

# CHAPTER 7

# Monitoring and Tracking Your Progress

Effective blood sugar management requires a proactive approach that involves continuous monitoring and tracking of your progress. This essential practice empowers you to make informed decisions, adapt your lifestyle as needed, and maintain stable blood sugar levels.

In this comprehensive guide, we will explore the importance of regular blood sugar monitoring and the value of keeping a food and activity journal in the context of blood sugar management.

## The Importance of Regular Blood Sugar Monitoring

Regular blood sugar monitoring is the cornerstone of effective diabetes management. Whether you have type 1, type 2 diabetes, prediabetes, or are simply striving for optimal blood sugar control, here's why monitoring is crucial:

1. Immediate Feedback: Monitoring provides immediate feedback on your blood sugar levels, allowing you to make timely adjustments to your treatment plan, diet, or exercise routine.

2. Individualized Insights: Everyone's response to food, exercise, and medication can vary. Monitoring helps you understand how your body reacts to specific factors, allowing you to tailor your management strategies accordingly.

3. Prevention of Highs and Lows: By tracking your blood sugar, you can catch and address both hyperglycemia (high blood sugar) and hypoglycemia (low blood sugar) before they become severe, reducing the risk of complications.

4. Medication Management: For those taking diabetes medications or insulin, monitoring helps ensure that you are taking the right dose at the right time, preventing dangerous fluctuations in blood sugar levels.

5. Improved A1c Control: Regular monitoring is directly linked to better HbA1c control, which provides a three-month average of your blood sugar levels. Consistently stable readings contribute to lower A1c levels.

6. Empowerment: Monitoring puts you in control of your health. It helps you identify patterns and trends, enabling you to make educated decisions about your diet, exercise, and medication regimen.

7. Health Awareness: Monitoring goes beyond just numbers. It promotes awareness of your overall health and encourages a proactive attitude toward managing your blood sugar.

# To effectively monitor your blood sugar

- Select the Right Device: Choose a glucose meter or continuous glucose monitoring (CGM) system that suits your needs and preferences.

- Follow a Schedule: Establish a routine for checking your blood sugar levels. Your healthcare provider can help determine the best times for testing.

- Log Results: Keep a record of your blood sugar readings, including date, time, and any relevant notes about meals, exercise, and medication.

- Examine Trends: Review your logs on a regular basis to find patterns or anomalies in your blood sugar levels. During your appointments, share this information with the medical professionals.

# Keeping a Food and Activity Journal

In addition to blood sugar monitoring, maintaining a detailed food and activity journal can provide valuable insights into how various factors impact your blood sugar levels. Here's how a food and activity journal can enhance your blood sugar management:

1. Dietary Awareness: Tracking your meals, snacks, and beverages allows you to recognize how different foods affect your blood sugar. You can identify which carbohydrates raise your levels significantly and adjust your diet accordingly.

2. Meal Timing: Recording when you eat helps you understand the relationship between meal timing and blood sugar fluctuations. This can guide you in planning meals and snacks to avoid sudden spikes or drops.

3. Portion Control: A journal can help you monitor portion sizes, preventing overeating and stabilizing post-meal blood sugar levels.

4. Exercise Insights: Record your physical activity, including type, duration, and intensity. This information helps you gauge the impact of exercise on your blood sugar and adjust your regimen accordingly.

5. Medication Management: If you take diabetes medication or insulin, noting the timing and dosage in your journal ensures you adhere to your prescribed regimen consistently.

6. Stress and Emotions: Documenting your emotional state and stress levels can reveal how these factors influence your blood sugar. Stress-reduction techniques can be implemented accordingly.

7. Pattern Recognition: Over time, your journal will reveal patterns and trends. For instance, you may notice that your blood sugar tends to spike after consuming certain foods or when you skip meals.

## To maintain an effective food and activity journal:

- Choose a Format: You can use a physical journal, a smartphone app, or a spreadsheet to log your information. Select a format that you're comfortable with and will consistently use.

- Be Detailed: Include specific details about your meals, portion sizes, and ingredients. Note the time of day, exercise type, duration, and any variations in your routine.

- Stay Consistent: Make journaling a daily habit. The more consistent you are, the more valuable your journal becomes for identifying trends and making adjustments.

- Review Regularly: Set aside time to review your journal entries. Look for correlations between your activities, meals, and blood sugar levels.

- Share with the Healthcare Team: Share your food and activity journal with your healthcare provider or diabetes educator during appointments. They can offer guidance based on your recorded data.

In conclusion, monitoring your blood sugar levels and keeping a detailed food and activity journal are fundamental practices in blood sugar management. These tools provide insights, empower you to make informed decisions, and help you maintain stable blood sugar levels over time. Remember that diabetes management is a dynamic process, and both monitoring and journaling are valuable allies in your journey toward better health and well-being.

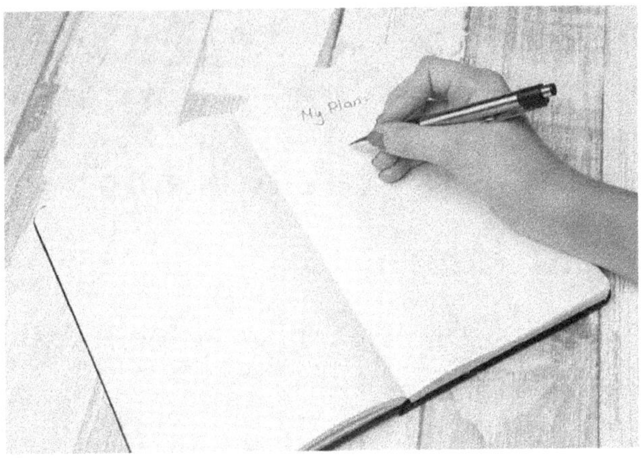

# CHAPTER 8

# Dealing with Challenges and Setbacks

Dealing with Challenges and Setbacks in Blood Sugar Management

Managing blood sugar levels is a continuous journey filled with both successes and challenges. It's common to encounter obstacles such as cravings, temptations, and plateaus along the way. Understanding how to navigate these challenges is crucial for maintaining stable blood sugar and overall well-being. In this comprehensive guide, we'll explore strategies to overcome cravings and temptations and cope with plateaus in blood sugar management.

# Overcoming Cravings and Temptations

Cravings and temptations can be powerful adversaries in the quest for better blood sugar control.

These desires for sugary or high-carbohydrate foods can disrupt your efforts. Here's how to conquer them:

1. Understand the Triggers:

Identify the triggers for your cravings. Is it stress, emotional factors, boredom, or certain situations? Recognizing these triggers can help you develop strategies to address them.

2. Balanced Meal Planning:

Plan balanced meals that include complex carbohydrates, fiber-rich foods, lean proteins, and healthy fats. This can help prevent sharp blood sugar spikes and minimize cravings.

3. Mindful Eating:

Practice mindful eating by paying attention to the taste, texture, and satisfaction of each bite. This can diminish the desire for excessive amounts of sweet or high-carb foods.

4. Keep Healthy Snacks on Hand:

Stock your pantry and refrigerator with healthy, blood-sugar-friendly snacks. Having options like fresh vegetables, nuts, and low-sugar fruits readily available can help curb cravings.

5. Stay Hydrated:

Thirst is sometimes confused with hunger. Always remember to drink plenty of water throughout the day to remain hydrated.

6. Manage Stress:

Stress can trigger cravings. Incorporate stress-reduction techniques like meditation, deep breathing exercises, or yoga into your routine to help manage stress and emotional eating.

7. Distract Yourself:

When a craving strikes, distract yourself with an engaging activity, like going for a walk, talking to a friend, or tackling a hobby. Often, cravings are temporary and will subside if you redirect your attention.

8. Gradual Reduction: If you're accustomed to high-sugar foods, consider reducing your sugar intake gradually. This can make it easier to adapt to a lower-sugar diet without feeling deprived.

9. Seek Support:

Join a support group or work with a healthcare professional or registered dietitian who specializes in blood sugar management. They are capable of providing guidance as well as assistance that can help you in managing urges.

## Coping with Plateaus:

Plateaus in blood sugar management occurs when your blood sugar levels remain relatively stable but stop improving. These plateaus can be frustrating, but there are strategies to break through them:

1. Reevaluate Your Routine:

Take a closer look at your diet, exercise, and medication regimen. Are you following your plan consistently? Plateaus can occur when there's a lack of adherence to your blood sugar management routine.

2. Adjust Your Diet:

Consider modifying your diet by making small changes.

This might involve adjusting portion sizes, changing the timing of your meals, or experimenting with different types of carbohydrates.

3. Modify Exercise Routine:

Review your exercise routine. Are you doing the same workouts repeatedly? Plateaus can happen when your body adapts to a consistent exercise routine. Try changing the intensity, duration, or type of exercise to challenge your body in new ways.

4. Monitor Blood Sugar Levels:

Regularly monitor your blood sugar levels, especially after meals and during different times of the day. This can provide insights into how your body responds to specific foods and activities.

5. Medication Adjustment:

If you're taking medication for blood sugar control, consult your healthcare provider. They may need to adjust their medication dosage or consider different medication options to break through a plateau.

## 6. Stay Patient and Positive:

Plateaus are a natural part of the blood sugar management journey. Stay patient and maintain a positive mindset. Celebrate the progress you've made and acknowledge that occasional plateaus are normal.

## 7. Set New Goals:

Reassess your goals. Once you've broken through a plateau, set new objectives to continue progressing in your blood sugar management journey.

## 8. Seek Professional Guidance:

Consider seeking guidance from a healthcare professional, such as an endocrinologist or diabetes educator. They can provide personalized recommendations and help you navigate plateaus effectively.

## 9. Support Network:

Lean on your support network, whether it's friends, family, or a diabetes support group. Sharing your experiences and challenges with others who understand can provide encouragement and motivation.

Dealing with challenges and setbacks in blood sugar management is an ongoing process that requires patience, perseverance, and adaptability. By implementing strategies to overcome cravings and temptations and coping with plateaus, you can maintain stable blood sugar levels and work toward your health and wellness goals. Remember that it's normal to encounter obstacles along the way, but with determination and support, you can continue on your path to better blood sugar control and overall health.

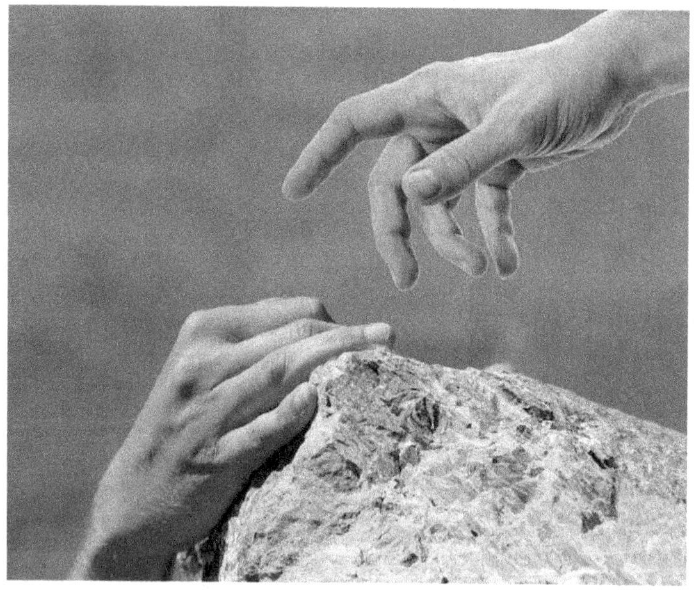

# Conclusion

In the journey towards better health and improved blood sugar management, the importance of a balanced and nutritious diet cannot be overstated. The Blood Sugar Diet Solution Cookbook has been meticulously crafted to provide you with a diverse array of delicious and blood sugar-friendly recipes that not only tantalize your taste buds but also support your well-being.

As we've explored throughout this cookbook, maintaining stable blood sugar levels is essential for overall health and can have a profound impact on preventing or managing conditions like diabetes. What you choose to put on your plate has a direct correlation to how your body functions, and by adopting the principles outlined in this cookbook, you've taken a significant step toward making informed and healthier choices.

Throughout these pages, you've discovered a treasure trove of recipes that not only prioritize low glycemic index ingredients but also champion the idea that eating well need not be boring or restrictive.

The recipes are a testament to the creativity and ingenuity of combining foods that are both nutritious and delightful. From hearty breakfasts to satisfying lunches, and from flavorful dinners to guilt-free desserts, these recipes offer a feast for your senses and a boon for your health.

In embracing these recipes, you've chosen to nourish your body with a rich tapestry of whole grains, lean proteins, an abundance of colorful vegetables, and healthy fats. You've learned how to create meals that provide sustained energy, curb cravings, and help prevent undesirable spikes and crashes in blood sugar levels.

You've also discovered how to use natural sweeteners judiciously and incorporate nutrient-dense superfoods into your daily diet.

Furthermore, you've taken a step towards embracing mindful eating and a holistic approach to health. It's not just about the food you eat but also about how you eat it. Savoring each bite, being in tune with your body's hunger and fullness cues, and cultivating a healthy relationship with food are all integral parts of maintaining balanced blood sugar levels and overall well-being.

As you continue your culinary journey with the recipes in this cookbook, remember that health is a lifelong endeavor. It's about making consistent, informed choices that support your body and mind. It's about finding joy in preparing and sharing nourishing meals with loved ones. It's about prioritizing self-care and self-love.

To make the most of the Blood Sugar Diet Solution Cookbook, consider consulting with a healthcare provider or registered dietitian who can offer personalized guidance tailored to your specific health needs and goals.

They can help you create a meal plan that aligns with your dietary preferences and health objectives, ensuring that you achieve optimal results in your blood sugar management journey.

In closing, we invite you to embrace the recipes in this cookbook not as restrictions but as opportunities to revitalize your health, invigorate your taste buds, and embark on a lifelong adventure towards balanced blood sugar levels and a vibrant, fulfilling life. Your health is an invaluable asset, and by making informed dietary choices, you're investing in a future brimming with vitality and well-being.

Here's to nourishing your health, one delicious and blood sugar-friendly meal at a time. Bon appétit!